Women
on Menopause

———

Women on Menopause

A PRACTICAL GUIDE TO A POSITIVE TRANSITION

---

by Anne Dickson and Nikki Henriques

HEALING ARTS PRESS
Rochester, Vermont

Healing Arts Press
One Park Street
Rochester, Vermont 05767

LIBRARY OF CONGRESS CATALOGING IN PUBLICATION DATA

Dickson, Anne, 1946–
Women on menopause.

Bibliography: p.
Includes index.
1. Menopause. 2. Menopause–Psychological aspects.
3. Women–Interviews. I. Henriques, Nikki. II. Title.
RG186.D53 1987   618.1'75   87–18043
ISBN 0–89281–237–0 (pbk.)

Printed and bound in the United States.

10 9 8 7 6 5 4 3 2 1

Healing Arts Press is a division of Inner Traditions International, Ltd.

Distributed to the book trade in the United States by Harper and Row
Publishers, Inc.
Distributed to the book trade in Canada by Book Center, Inc., Montreal,
Quebec
Distributed to the health food trade in Canada by Alive Books, Toronto and
Vancouver

Contents

Acknowledgements

———

WE are indebted to the following people, the women who agreed to be interviewed about their experience of the menopause: Dot, Olive, Barbara, Madeleine, Linda, Sue, Brenda, Shirley, Mary, Alix, Grania, Antonia, Rita, Jayne, and Doris, who contributed in a major way to the material in this book.

The gynecologists and Menopause Clinic Nurses: Dr. Patricia Last, Mr. Nicholas Siddle, Mr. John McGarry, Mr. Himansu Basu; family planning expert Dr. Pramilla Senanayake; and nurses Lysette Butler and Julie Endacott, all of whom gave their time to be interviewed and whose professional experience and insight has been invaluable.

We are especially grateful to Misha Norland, homeopathic practitioner and teacher, for introducing us to the principles of homeopathy and for taking the time to prepare a self-help section on homeopathy for this book.

We would also like to thank Mrs. Ann Warren-Davis, medical herbalist, for her time and information.

We would also like to express our thanks to Jayne, who, apart from being interviewed, generously gave us access to her considerable library of menopausal literature.

Last, we are indebted to the British Medical Association Press Office for help and library facilities.

Foreword

———

THE menopause is not natural. A century ago it was natural for the majority of women to be dead before they would have experienced the trials and tribulations, or even joys, of the menopause. Those who survived had other things to worry about than the cessation of their periods. It certainly was not a topic for conversation then, as it seems to be now.

In the West, the baby girl celebrating her first birthday today does so in the confident expectation that she will live well into her mid-seventies. Today, a woman will live some twenty-five years after her reproductive–though not her sexual–life is complete: a third of a lifetime.

It is hardly surprising that with the comparative novelty of the menopause experience, information and misinformation abound. Attention is variously focused on the medical, social, and emotional problems that can occur at this time in a woman's life, but all these aspects are closely if not inextricably interwoven. No sensible or realistic person, whether doctor or layperson, should try to separate them. While symptoms can be treated by medicines, a simplistic approach such as this is unlikely to be completely rewarding in the complex situation of the female menopause.

There are many books about the menopause written by authors with either personal or professional experience. The present authors have neither: they are not doctors, nor are they old enough to have had experience of their own menopause – although, as you may know from their previous book, *Women on Hysterectomy*, Nikki has herself had a hysterectomy. The authors are, however, skilled and interested observers, and by drawing on the experiences of menopausal women from a wide variety of backgrounds and balancing these experiences against the currently received wisdom, they have produced an essentially practical and at the same time personal guide for women entering the climacteric. Not only are women's attitudes sampled, but so are the attitudes of some of the doctors who see the small proportion of menopausal women who are referred to specialist clinics.

At the present time, few women take medication to help their menopausal symptoms. The vast majority "grin and bear it" or claim to have no symptoms worth bothering about. This book will help readers discover the large variety of normality that exists at the time of the menopause. It will also help them to make an informed decision about whether or not to use hormone replacement therapy or even nonhormonal treatments to alleviate their symptoms. They will be enormously heartened by sharing the experiences recorded in this book.

Patricia Last
Fellow of the Royal College of Surgeons,
Fellow of the Royal College of Obstetricians and Gynecologists

Introduction
(Is She Still a Lady?)

———

RUMOR has it that the menopausal woman is deranged, even criminal:

> "I thought I was supposed to feel absolutely awful during it, that it was a dreadful period in a woman's life, because of the descriptions I'd heard women say about other women. You know, 'Betty's been absolutely mad ever since the change.' Those sorts of vague and horrible things." (*Geraldine*)

> "I can remember growing up and the almost hushed tones of 'You know, it's the change,' said with some foreboding, as if *the change* could be Jekyll and Hyde, or God knows what! There was great weight to the words 'the change' even though I was only a kid." (*Bea*)

> "I'd heard as a child this is the time you can go mental–everyone knows people who went mad; all sorts of things happen to them, even dropping down dead in the street, all due to the menopause." (*Doreen*)

> "I used to think about shoplifting. All the people you read about say they didn't know that they were doing it, so I used to be very careful about paying–keeping my hands together." (*Maureen*)

1

And if you need reassurance, it's preferable to avoid the clinical definition, of which this is just one example:

> The menopause signifies that a woman has climbed to a higher rung in her ascent up the ladder of life—the climacteric. Ovarian function subsides, estrogen production declines and menstrual flow ceases; she is now freed from the responsibilities, the stresses, the hazards and the trials and tribulations of childbirth—but at a price. For many, the effects of estrogen deprivation are devastating: for a fortunate few the damage is minimal, the scars only slightly visible. (R. B. Greenblatt, Retired Professor of Endocrinology, Medical College of Georgia, USA: *British Journal of Sexual Medicine*, December, 1981.)

Not one positive word for the whole of a woman's reproductive experience! Hardly an encouragement to welcome the menopause with open arms. So how do we react when it happens?

"I didn't expect anything much to happen; that's why it was a big shock, because quite a lot did happen. It all took me by surprise, because I thought I knew my body quite well." (*Angela*)

"A tremendous relief, that I wouldn't have to bother with my diaphragm anymore. That's the nicest thing." (*Brenda*)

"Sadness and a kind of poignancy, thinking, gosh, times are changing. I'm getting older. . . ." (*Bea*)

"I anticipated it would happen fairly early, as I was a late starter. But I really didn't think about it; I just knew it was going to happen one day." (*Doreen*)

"I thought I was going to be one of the lucky ones who got away with it. I didn't get there till fifty-five, and I was thinking, 'This is never going to happen to me!'" (*Anne*)

"I sailed through all my pregnancies without problems and then for all this to happen just because all this was ending seemed so unfair and so untrue." (*Rosie*)

"I was sad, actually—a certain feeling of loss about it. Silly, isn't it?" (*Sheila*)

"In cultures where marriage at thirteen or fourteen is common, followed by numerous pregnancies at frequent intervals, women find reaching menopause a great relief. They say, 'Thank God, I reached my menopause. I will never have to go through more pregnancies again'. . . ." (*Snanayake*). So these women look upon menopause very positively.

Statistics state that 25 percent of all women pass through their menopause without noticing it, 25 percent suffer quite severely, and the remaining 50 percent are aware of some menopausal changes to a greater or lesser extent.

Maybe you are one of that 25 percent who notices nothing other than an end to your periods. But the majority of women will notice and feel something: they may suffer acute and chronic stress, and many will seek help in the form of medical intervention to alleviate symptoms.

We interviewed women from a variety of backgrounds, but we did not attempt to research cross-cultural attitudes to the menopause, and we have limited our brief to menopause as it affects women in western culture. The women were:*

Angela: Fifty-six, four children, psychotherapist and poet.
Anne: Fifty-seven, one child, social worker.
Bea: Forty-six, two children, community administrator.
Brenda: Fifty-four, one child, justice of the peace.
Caroline: Sixty-seven, retired senior dental assistant.
Diana: Sixty, two children, beauty therapist.
Doreen: Fifty-two, personnel manager.
Geraldine: Fifty-eight, three children, counselor and teacher.
Jo: Forty-four, three children, author and teacher.
Lisa: Forty-four, two children, teacher and writer.
Mary: Sixty-three, retired hospital matron.
Maureen: Sixty-three, one child, retired airlines administrator.
Rosie: Fifty-two, five children, retired merchandise buyer.
Sheila: Fifty-three, two children, senior nurse tutor.
Sylvia: Forty-four, four children, writer and peace-worker.

We are aware that many women have no interest in understanding what goes on inside their bodies and would rather remain

*We have changed the names of the women interviewed to maintain confidentiality.

ignorant. It does involve an effort to find out and to understand what's happening, and we hope the following chapters offer a comprehensive and above all *positive* guide to what can happen during the menopause, why it happens, and what you can do about it.

Anne Dickson and Nikki Henriques

1

Before and After

———

"WHAT does the menopause mean to you?" we asked. In a way, it's relatively easy to answer this question. To Geraldine, it meant "cessation of periods"; to Caroline, "ending of fertility." Like most answers, these correctly associate menopause with the end of menstruation. But other responses indicate wider issues:

"The change—another steppingstone." (*Doreen*)

"A transition from feeling young to feeling older." (*Angela*)

"Change of one's body altogether." (*Mary*)

"A bloody nuisance." (*Anne*)

The menopause—which literally means the last menstrual period—can be identified in retrospect and is a fixed point in every woman's life. In contrast, the description and explanation of the years before the actual menopause and after that event are complicated and impossible to define precisely.

The changes that occur during these years are gradual and long-lasting. They are physiological changes, psychological changes, and often social changes. There is no clearly marked beginning and no definite end to the menopausal years. All that we know is that these years follow certain stages and that within those stages there is a wide range of variation.

The normal span of the entire menopausal transition varies from one to five years, with most women experiencing about two years and a minority as long as fifteen years. The average age at the last period is fifty-one, but it is still considered normal if this occurs anytime between forty-five and fifty-five.

According to popular belief, a woman will follow the same pattern of menopause as her mother, and although this may sometimes be true, there is no scientific proof that it is generally so. Up to now, the evidence points to tentative links with the following:

- *Smoking*: If you are or have been a heavy smoker, then you are more likely to experience an early menopause.
- *Height*: Tall women often experience a later menopause.
- *Marital status*: It's possible that married women experience menopause later than women without a partner.
- *Children*: There also appears to be a link between a late menopause and pregnancy after the age of forty. Women without children often have a later menopause than those with children.

Although these links are interesting, they do not allow us to make predictions with any real certainty.

A woman's body, in particular her reproductive system, is the central agent in this process of change. Although our physical changes are complex and therefore difficult to understand, it's important to have a basic knowledge of what's happening in order to allay anxiety and deal more carefully and wisely with the changes that do occur, so that we can pass through the transition positively.

Cycles

To grasp the essence of these changes, it's helpful to think in terms of cycles. The menopausal years mark the gradual ending of a woman's reproductive cycle. At birth a baby girl is born with an average of 400,000 eggs in her ovaries ready to fulfill the adult function of reproduction. The supply of eggs diminishes through-out her life, so that at puberty her ovaries will contain about 75,000 eggs, and by the time she's forty, about 5,000.

At puberty the brain triggers hormonal changes, which result in a girl's beginning her menstrual cycle; the first bleeding is her first period. From then on until menopause, her menstrual cycle will normally continue every month unless interrupted by pregnancy.

The most obvious marker of the menstrual cycle is the monthly bleeding, but physiologically the bleeding is only one small aspect. The cycle of hormonal change that occurs in the weeks preceding menstruation and continues through menstruation and afterward is far more important. Bleeding is simply the mechanical response of the womb to the hormonal changes. This monthly bleeding is the most easily identifiable event in the normal menstrual cycle, and for many women, as they approach menopause, the first sign that something is changing is the irregularity of this pattern.

In order to understand the effects of hormonal changes, we need first to understand what a hormone is.

What Is a Hormone?

Hormones are substances that stimulate organs into action. They are produced by certain glands, and travel through the body in the blood. These glands are controlled by the hypothalamus, a central mechanism in the brain that acts as a monitor of all the hormonal levels throughout the body. The glands that secrete the hormones are the *pituitary* gland, which lies at the base of the brain; the *thyroid*, which lies at the base of the throat; the *adrenal* gland, on top of the kidneys; and the *gonad* glands, situated in the ovaries of women and the testes of men.

The task of a hormone is to stimulate or inhibit activity in target areas of the body. As it is secreted a hormone travels to that area, where it is absorbed and sets off a chain reaction.

The hormones concerned in the reproductive cycle are *estrogens*, *progestogens*, and *androgens*. The principle sites of secretion of these three groups of hormones are, respectively, the ovaries in women, the testes in men, and the adrenal glands of both women and men.

These glands all manufacture estrogens and androgens, but in different amounts. In addition, these hormones are produced in other places in the body such as the liver, the muscles, and the fatty tissue.

Estrogen

This is the most frequently mentioned hormone in relation to menopause. In fact, estrogen doesn't refer to one single hormone but to a group of hormones responsible for producing female sexual characteristics. The most powerful kind of estrogen is estradiol. This can be broken down and "diluted" to a weaker form, estrone, which in turn may be broken down to form the weakest kind of estrogen, estriol. All these three estrogens occur naturally in the body.

Estrogens are specifically responsible for certain changes in the menstrual cycle, which will be described in the next section. They also affect the woman's body in general ways. They promote cell growth and repair in a woman's genitals, maintain the healthy condition of the vaginal walls, and regulate the vaginal mucus, which acts as a defense against infection.

Estrogens are also responsible for the formation of the duct system in the breast, and the formation of fatty tissue. They act as a protection to the bones, because they help to increase the retention of calcium, and also they act on the blood itself to decrease cholesterol.

Why we need estrogen:
- Stimulates growth and blood circulation in all genital areas: vulva, vagina, and uterus.
- Increases cervical secretions.
- Repairs and thickens endometrium.
- Increases muscular activity of the fallopian tubes.
- Affects production of egg sac stimulating hormones (FSH) in hypothalamus in brain.

- Affects breast development: pigmentation of nipple area and breast duct system.
- Improves blood circulation.
- Helps retain calcium in bones.
- Contributes to female hair distribution, vocal pitch, physical shape, and stature.
- Increases libido.

Progesterone

This hormone is one of the group called progestogens. The main function of this group is the preparation of the womb as a home for the fertilized egg, and the maintenance of pregnancy. In the middle of the menstrual cycle, when the egg is released from the egg sac (ovulation), the empty egg sac transforms itself into a yellowish mass of tissue called the *corpus luteum*. This is where the progesterone is produced. Although its main function occurs during pregnancy, our chief concern with progesterone during the menopause is that it counteracts some of the effects of estrogen.

Why we need progesterone:
- Prepares body for pregnancy.
- Thickens the endometrium.
- Reduces cervical secretions.
- Reduces uterine wall muscular activity.
- Inhibits production of the luteinizing hormone (LH); prevents ovulation.
- Contributes to water and salt retention in body.
- Stimulates growth of alveoli (milk-secreting cells) in the breast tissues.

Androgens

This group of hormones promotes the development of male sexual characteristics in men, as estrogens promote female characteristics in women, although men have some estrogens just as women have some androgens. The principle androgen is testosterone, which in men is produced primarily in the testes. In a woman, half of her testosterone is secreted by the adrenal gland and the other half is converted from another substance (androstenedione), also secreted by the adrenal gland and the ovary. This means that a woman's major source of androgens is her adrenal glands.

Androgens stimulate growth, encourage muscular development, and help to strengthen bones by increasing the retention of calcium.

Two other major hormones will concern us. These are produced in the pituitary gland and are called follicle stimulating hormone (FSH), so called because it stimulates the growth of the eggs in their follicles, or sacs, and luteinizing hormone (LH), so called because it transforms the empty follicle after the egg has been released into the *corpus luteum*.

The Menstrual Cycle

The best way to begin to understand the hormonal changes leading up to the menopause is to first understand what happens throughout our reproductive cycle. Once we have grasped a normal pattern, we can better understand what happens as the pattern changes and as the cycle comes to an end.

The menstrual cycle can be divided into five phases.

1. *The menstrual phase*: Days 1–5.
   The first day of bleeding is Day 1 because it marks the simultaneous ending of one cycle and the beginning of the next.
2. *The follicular phase*: Days 6–12.
   The FSH arrives at the ovaries to stimulate growth of the new follicles. As they grow they produce estrogen; as the level of estrogen in the bloodstream rises it signals to the brain that there is enough; so, with the brain acting as monitor, the FSH level drops.

   The follicles need to protect themselves against this drop in FSH, so they absorb as much as they can, but as there's not enough to go around, only one eventually survives and the others decline. The surviving follicle continues to produce estrogen, so that the level rises sharply by Day 7 and peaks toward the end of this phase, when the size of the surviving follicle is at its largest.

The FSH levels, meanwhile, remain low. The follicles that stop growing don't simply die away; they continue to produce a little estrogen and small amounts of androgens.

3. *The ovulatory phase*: Days 13–15.

On Day 13, the level of the estrogen has reached its critical level and is maintained for several hours; this signals to the brain the next important stage–the release of LH. The surge of LH into the bloodstream causes the surviving follicle to burst and expel the mature egg; this is called ovulation and occurs at about Day 15. The egg (ovum) is then transported for fertilization toward the uterus by the contractions of the fallopian tube.

We are now in mid-cycle.

4. *The luteal phase*: Days 16–22.

Under the influence of LH, an important process of transformation occurs. The now empty follicle reforms into a yellowish structure on the surface of the ovary, called the *corpus luteum*. The *corpus luteum* is responsible for producing progesterone, which continues to rise throughout the rest of this and the next phase. The progesterone is responsible for the preparation of the womb for pregnancy. The endometrium (lining of the womb) thickens with the increased blood supply, providing a potential plush environment for the fertilized egg. If fertilization takes place, another hormone is released; if the egg remains unfertilized, the luteal phase is brought to an end and the *corpus luteum* disintegrates.

5. *The premenstrual phase*; Days 23–28.

With the disintegration of the *corpus luteum*, there is a rapid decline in estrogen and progesterone over about four days. The effect can be dramatic, possibly affecting moods, appetite, balance, and mobility. The endometrium is particularly affected by the withdrawal of progesterone. The blood vessels, which have been supplying the womb in preparation for the fertilized egg, now go into spasm and contract. The walls break, hemorrhage occurs, and the lining comes away from the womb and is shed. Thus, the period begins and we're back to Day 1.

While the levels of progesterone and estrogen are falling during the premenstrual phase, the FSH is slowly rising and going on to initiate the growth of a new set of follicles, thus starting off a whole new cycle. In this way, each cycle overlaps with the next.

The menstrual cycle is like a clock, with the ovaries acting as the timing mechanism. The cycle is determined and maintained by the rhythm of the ovaries. It is the rhythm of each ovary that causes subtle yet significant changes in the hormone levels. The key to the menstrual cycle is ovulation; once ovulation has occurred, the events leading to menstruation will proceed.

The early cycles of puberty and the late cycles of menopause can occur without ovulation. This is because in puberty the eggs are not mature enough, whereas in menopausal years the eggs have been used up or have naturally disintegrated.

The ovaries have a limited lifespan. It is fascinating that regardless of the social and environmental changes through history, the ovarian timing mechanism stops at the same point. A century ago, for example, a woman's life expectancy was on average, forty-eight years. Now she has a life expectancy in the West, on average, of seventy-five years. Yet, even though life expectancy is longer, the age of menopause—that is, a woman's last menstruation—has not extended. It still happens at about fifty for the vast majority of women.

Physical Changes

Now that their work is done, the ovaries gradually slow down and eventually stop altogether. This process means that our hormonal levels will be changed. As the ovary is the principal producer of estrogen, it is the drop in this hormone in particular that affects different parts of the body.

As we saw earlier, hormones affect the body in different ways, so when levels change after the last period, the effects of these changes can be detected in various ways. *The rate and extent of these changes vary enormously from woman to woman.*

Genitals

On the inside, the reproductive organs gradually become smaller. On the outside, the inner and outer lips become less pronounced, and the pubic hair becomes thinner. The elasticity of the pelvic muscles can also be reduced. The inner membrane can become less moist; and without lubrication, the vagina is less protected from infection.

Breasts

The breasts can lose fullness and firmness in response to reduced estrogen stimulation of the tissue.

Skin

There is evidence to show that falling estrogen affects the skin, but it's difficult to distinguish which changes occur with old age and which are specific to the menopause, because skin changes occur in both men and women at this time and throughout the rest of their lives. Lack of estrogen is thought to increase dryness of the skin because the ability to retain water is diminished.

Bones

The density of bones declines after the menopause, partly because estrogen is no longer at the level to help store calcium in the bones. In some women this is believed to lead in later life to an increased risk of osteoporosis, a condition in which the bones become markedly less dense and therefore less strong and more liable to break easily. (See Chapter 3.)

Blood

After the menopause, levels of cholesterol rise because estrogen has previously protected the body against this. Until the menopause, women are comparatively free of coronary heart disease; afterward, the risk of heart disease in women is increased rapidly in comparison with the risk in a man of the same age.

The Change in Perspective

Reading through a list of the physical changes associated with the end of the reproductive cycle, you could be forgiven for thinking "Is there life after menopause?" The truth is that there *are* changes. Our bodies are changing all the time, and when one important aspect of our lives comes to an end, there are bound to be physical repercussions. But we emphasize that these changes vary with individual women.

It is nothing but a direct reflection of our culture if these changes are regarded as negative. If we lived in a society less obsessed with youth and physical beauty, these changes would not be regarded as symptoms of a terminal disease. Instead, they would be seen as one natural part of the whole: as one integral aspect of an extraordinary and quite miraculous cycle in a woman's life.

2

Signs

———

THE whole period of transition from our fully reproductive years to the nonreproductive phase of our lives is technically called the climacteric. So, when we discuss menopause we take into consideration the experience of the changes *leading up to* our last period (technically called the perimenopausal phase) and the changes *following* the last period (the postmenopausal phase).

Indications

What are the indications or signs that we are undergoing a change connected with the menopause? The most obvious reference point is menstruation. The majority of women interviewed noticed an irregularity of some kind in their monthly cycles. The irregular pattern is most easily understood in terms of the gradual winding down of the ovaries, which begin to slow down as early as ten years before the menopause.

In the last chapter we described ovulation as the key event in the menstrual cycle, after which you can expect the other hormonal events to follow. Before the menopause itself, the ovary slows down, and so the production of estrogen falls. The subtle rela-

15

tionship between the hormone monitor (the hypothalamus) and the two hormone producers (the pituitary and the ovary) changes gradually, bringing the reproductive cycle to an end.

While this relationship changes, our bodies can experience some chaos: the hormone monitor can signal production of FSH, following its usual monthly program, which would normally stimulate the ovaries to produce enough estrogen to feed back to the brain to lower the FSH. But now what happens is that the ovaries can't produce enough estrogen for the feedback system to work. Therefore, no egg is produced, or if it is, it may not be released. Without ovulation, progesterone is not produced, so we do not bleed.

Instead of one phase of the cycle lasting a few days, weeks or months can pass until the next phase is signaled. It takes time for the monitor to adjust to the new situation, and this is why one of the most recognizable signs of an imminent menopause is irregular menstruation.

"Usually a slackening off of periods or irregular periods, missing one and then being regular for two or three months, and then missing a period for six months and coming back for a couple of months. Anything with that kind of pattern is normal." (*Last*)

"The commonest problem I see is a woman who has one period which is light, then a long gap then a period which goes on and on and is very heavy, and which distresses her." (*McGarry*)

A wide variety of patterns was reported by our interviewees:

"That's the first thing; I didn't have a period. It gradually got less and less, lighter and lighter, but went on regularly until it finally petered out altogether." (*Maureen*)

"The first thing, my periods began to get irregular, some of them annoyingly heavy, but nothing too bad. They seemed to finish for a whole eight months, there was nothing, and I thought 'Ah, it's over.' Then suddenly it was back again." (*Angela*)

"It didn't come for five months, then came back half-heartedly, then it stopped and I haven't had one since." (*Sylvia*)

"I didn't think about it until my cycle changed. Instead of getting scanty and further apart, I was completely in reverse. Much heavier and much more often. That went on for three years." (*Mary*)

"I only had a period every other month and then I stopped suddenly. A whole year afterwards—I remember distinctly; we were on holiday in Greece—I went to the toilet and couldn't believe it. It was very difficult trying to buy Tampax on a Greek island. I never had another one after." (*Brenda*)

"They are longer and heavier and I can get enormous clots sometimes." (*Bea*)

"I noticed my periods diminishing, but it was never a problem." (*Doreen*)

One woman we spoke to realized only in retrospect that she'd been through the menopause, because her menstrual cycle had never followed a regular pattern.

"I was so irregular all through my life, that it didn't worry me that I went a couple of months with nothing. When I'd gone six months with nothing happening, I thought, 'Well, that must be the end.' I never had any flooding or anything at all." (*Caroline*)

It's quite usual at this time, when periods are becoming irregular, for women to notice symptoms associated with the premenstrual phase of the cycle, when physical and emotional stress can be quite acute, even though the period itself fails to arrive.

"I started getting very emotionally upset and finding a tremendous drain of confidence, and I found this was happening once a month and getting very severe." (*Anne*)

"The feeling that your period is coming, an awful feeling of being blown up, and pain, and dragging, then nothing. Then that would disappear and perhaps return a month later." (*Mary*)

"My periods started fluctuating, and then the bloating began and I could see my breasts, getting bigger every day and really painful." (*Rosie*)

"My breasts began to get particularly tender, so sensitive that I could hardly bear to have clothes against them. It was unusual to have them as tender as that for such a long time." (*Bea*)

A woman's experience of menstruation is highly individual, and so too will be her experience of menopausal changes. Although the pattern of irregularity will vary woman to woman—as to the length of time between periods, the heaviness of flow, and the number of days of flow—the most common way for menstruation to stop is *irregularly*.

It's important to distinguish between this kind of irregular pattern and abnormal bleeding. The term "abnormal bleeding" includes hemorrhaging, which is a flow of blood that exceeds that of a heavy period. It also refers to staining outside the menstrual period or to excessive frequency of periods. These may not be indications that anything is seriously wrong, but it is always worth checking out with your doctor.

"Irregular periods that occur at regular intervals, or normal periods that occur at irregular intervals are acceptable. But spotting all over the place is not." (*Last*)

We should add that menstruation may cease earlier than the menopause for all sorts of reasons, a very common one being some form of acute stress. It is not unusual for a woman in her forties to assume that if her periods stop, she must be menopausal, when the cause may be elsewhere.

Anne put her irregular periods and feelings of dread down to menopause when she was forty-six, and then later discovered that it had to do with the stress of anticipating her brother's release from prison. Her periods returned normally, and subsequently stopped when she reached the menopause six years later. Lisa also expected her periods to stop early because she had been told that her mother had stopped menstruating in her early forties. But like Anne, Lisa found that the reason was stress—in her case, after a miscarriage.

As long as you have even part of a normally functioning ovary, you will experience your menopause at your natural time.

If both ovaries cease to function because of disease or surgical removal—for example, hysterectomy—the menopause may be experienced earlier.

Premature Menopause

Although the ovaries eventually stop working in every woman, some women experience premature ovarian failure. This may be because they were born without ovaries in the first place, or it may be that their ovaries are present but that they never started ovulating, or again, it may be that this particular gland stops working in the same way as any other gland can stop working.

One nurse we interviewed told us that this group of women has very specific needs. "They tend to be in their twenties or early thirties and feel freakish and isolated, having to deal with problems of powerlessness and absolute infertility. Their experience of menopause is obviously different from that of the older menopausal woman, who has usually had her family and is psychologically more ready to deal with physical changes." (*Endacott*)

This nurse did in fact start a self-help group for these very special young women, and she reported that it helped them to meet and identify with others in the same situation. Many of them had already developed a positive attitude, some putting their energy into adopting a child, and others into a career.

Hysterectomy

A hysterectomy can be one of two kinds: subtotal, which means that only the body of the womb has been removed, or total, which means that the body of the womb and the cervix have been removed.

Sadly, since the cervix is now recognized as a possible cancer site in later life, its removal is automatic unless (a) you specifically request that it be left in place, (b) it is healthy, or (c) the surgeon agrees to your request.

Leaving the cervix intact makes it much easier for the surgeon because it is unnecessary to first cut into and then stitch the top of the vagina. Consequently, the delicate and accident-prone ureter is avoided.

If you express the wish to have your cervix retained, and if you agree to annual cervical smears, there's no reason why the cervix shouldn't be retained. It's just somewhat unusual.

It is always important to ask your surgeon whether or not your ovaries were removed when you have had a hysterectomy.

If a woman has a hysterectomy before her menopause and her ovaries are left intact, she will not experience the menopause until her natural time, because as long as the ovaries are present they continue to ensure that the necessary supply of estrogen is produced.

The other hormonal changes will continue in their usual way. That's why after hysterectomy, women can still recognize the symptoms they previously knew to be part of the menstrual cycle, such as breast tenderness, mood changes, and water retention.

The only thing that is different is that there will be no more bleeding, because the uterus is no longer there. Obviously, then, irregular bleeding patterns will not be relevant to a woman without her uterus. But she may still experience some of the other menopausal symptoms described in the following chapter.

Ovariectomy

At the time of hysterectomy, one or both ovaries and fallopian tubes may be removed. The ovaries are invariably removed if they show any signs of disease. They are also removed at the age of menopause or just afterward, as they are no longer making any significant amounts of hormones. Once the ovaries have been removed, of course, they cannot become cancerous, and many surgeons believe it is an advantage to carry out this procedure at the time of menopause.

If your ovaries are removed before your natural menopause, your experience will be different: you will usually experience menopausal symptoms. If your ovaries are removed when your natural menopause is imminent, the symptoms are not quite so severe. That's why a woman who has her ovaries removed in her twenties or thirties will almost certainly be prescribed an estrogen substitute, in order to avoid symptoms of premature aging, and she will be advised to take it for the rest of her life.

We have written more fully about hysterectomy in our book *Women on Hysterectomy: How Long Before I Can Hang-Glide?*, published by Thorsons Publishing Group, Wellingborough.

3

Experience

———

THE most frequently reported menopausal symptom is the hot flush, or flash. It is believed to be experienced to some degree at some point by 75–85 percent of women.

Technically described as a "vasomotor disturbance," the hot flush is the result of chemical and hormonal changes taking place in the body. Suddenly the brain perceives that the body has overheated, and initiates a series of changes in the nervous system that cause the body to try to cool itself down. To do this, the blood vessels near the skin surface dilate, and blood pours through the vessels, bringing heat to the skin. In this way the heat radiates outward, the hot skin perspires, and evaporation of the moisture cools the body down again.

This process happens normally when the body becomes overheated. For some reason as yet unknown, during our menopausal years, communication between the skin and the brain can be temporarily disturbed. Even if a woman doesn't feel herself to be hot, she can experience this sudden flush of heat to her skin – her face, neck, and chest feel hot – followed immediately afterward by perspiration, shivering, and a chilled feeling.

Hot flushes are usually experienced during the day. At night they take the form of night sweats – you wake up because of the heat and will often have to throw off the bedclothes for immediate relief. The frequency of hot flushes and night sweats varies enormously from one a day or one an hour to several times an hour. They also vary in duration from one minute to about four minutes.

The "Flushing Band"

This disturbance is known to be associated with low estrogen levels in the bloodstream, but this is not the full explanation. Hot flushes and night sweats are also associated with an increase of FSH, the pituitary hormone, in the blood, but whereas raised levels of this hormone occur in every woman, not every woman flushes. Because of the extraordinary range and variations of the experience of hot flushes and night sweats, medical research cannot pinpoint their cause, although the association with low estrogen levels does mean that estrogen is frequently administered to women if this particular symptom becomes very severe. Progestogens also reduce flushes and may be preferred as medication by some women.

One explanation of the incidence of hot flushes is the "flushing band" theory. Imagine a band with the top edge indicating a high level of estrogen, and the lower edge, a low level of estrogen. In between the two levels, it is believed hot flushes occur, so that if a woman's estrogen level is above or below the band limits, she will not experience hot flushes. However, the extent of the band varies from woman to woman. If this theory is correct, it could explain why some women have flushes and others don't, depending on the individual woman's level of estrogen. It could also explain not only why a woman can experience flushing phases but why flushes can stop, presumably when the estrogen level in her body has naturally fallen below the band.

When Do Hot Flushes Start?

They can begin in the years preceding the end of menstruation and can continue for several years afterward. One of the gynecologists interviewed suggested that 80 percent of women who experience hot flushes do so for a period of about two years, with the remaining 20 percent experiencing them for longer than that, perhaps for as long as fifteen years.

Ten of the fifteen women we interviewed experienced hot flushes to a greater or lesser extent, and eight of them also had night sweats.

"I can be sitting here just lovely and cool and comfortable, then all of a sudden, your whole body just burns on fire, from your head down. The perspiration just trickles off you and your body's all sticky and clammy." (*Brenda*)

"Out of the blue, from your neck down to your waist. I always felt conscious of a scarlet neck, but I had more sweating than flushes. In the night I'd wake up wringing wet and have to get up and towel myself down." (*Mary*)

"It's very uncomfortable, prickly all over, and you come out in perspiration. One minute you're hot, and suddenly you find perspiration trickling down your face, even on a cool day." (*Sheila*)

"I didn't have a red face. I didn't blush at all, so nobody knew I was having them." (*Maureen*)

"It was mostly in bed, suddenly having to throw off the bedclothes and things." (*Sylvia*)

"I just felt hot all over. I used to call them my 'breakouts' because that's exactly what they are." (*Doreen*)

"It's different from a feeling of just getting hot. There is a feeling almost as if you're feeling a bit sick as well. It comes from the inside." (*Anne*)

One of the reasons why women seek help to alleviate this symptom is the distress and embarrassment it causes them.

"I've been in the most awful places, and it's happened, and you feel terribly conscious that everyone's looking at you. You feel awful and the next moment it's gone." (*Brenda*)

Brenda took a course of treatment to help. (See more in Chapter 7.) Many women, on the other hand, prefer to stick it out; one example is Maureen, who at the time of the interview had experienced flushes for twelve years. She did not wish to take pills, and therefore learned to live with the flushes.

" 'I'll just put up with it for a few years,' I thought. But those few years have gone on and on! You get to know what clothes to wear, you don't wear anything tight around your neck, don't wear trousers on a hot day, you just know what to do." (*Maureen*)

Many women learn the benefit of appropriate clothing.

"I find it a great help to wear loose clothing. Rather than putting on slim-fitting clothes, I tend to wear loose blouses and skirts, probably a size larger than I need to." (*Doreen*)

As Maureen pointed out, it is important not to wear anything too tight around the neck, to avoid scarves and high-necked sweaters. Maureen bought herself an old-fashioned fan, which she took everywhere with her. Any very hot drink can trigger a flush, and substances like alcohol or curried food that make people hot in normal circumstances can often make life much worse for a menopausal woman.

Another contributing factor to flushing is believed to be body weight. The reason is that higher estrogen levels are associated with fatty tissue; therefore, extremely thin women can have less circulating estrogen and could be more vulnerable to hot flushes.

Both the weather and stress of any kind are also contributory factors. In hot weather a woman is more susceptible to flushes, and stress exacerbates the whole experience. Stress stimulates the adrenal glands, causing extra hormonal activity, which in turn sparks off a flushing response.

After nine years' experience of flushing, Doreen said, "I notice if I get particularly stressed about things or emotional about something, it activates it. I try very hard to control stress, anyway. But because I'm an emotional person it's extremely difficult. But I do find I'm able to control the breakouts in a way. I try to keep calm, not rush around, and stand by the open window or a fan and basically cool down."

Palpitations

Five of our interviewees said that palpitations often occurred with the hot flush. This symptom is associated with the menopause, but there is as yet no known cause.

"There were quite a few palpitations; they often come out in the night associated with the flush, so there'd be a terrific surge of flushing, energy, and my heart beating very fast." (*Angela*)

Headaches

Sometimes headaches are described as a symptom of the menopause because they belong in the same category as flushes and palpitations. Some women experience severe migraine-like headaches, but others find that their headaches actually *decrease*. One woman reported a bizarre individual experience, which she found terribly distressing.

"I was convinced with all these queer feelings in my head, I had a brain tumor. The only way that I can describe it was that it felt like an octopus was inside my head. The body was there and each tentacle would press, trying to get out. My throat felt restricted; my vision blurred; I felt as though I was deaf." (*Rosie*)

She never learned the cause of this sensation.

Other Changes

After the hot flushes and related physiological experiences, the next broad category of change takes place in the rate at which our blood cells repair and grow.

Genital Changes

The decline in estrogen supply at menopause affects the rate of cell growth in all our tissues and body organs. Many women first become aware of this change in their genitals, which is described clinically as "genital atrophy." It simply indicates a *gradual* breakdown in tissue, and the inevitable effects of aging will begin to show. For example, the skin of the vagina and the vulva thins, and the pubic hair turns gray.

These changes are continuous, starting in our late forties or fifties, the most extreme aging effects being visible in very elderly women (a parallel process occurs in elderly men, too!). We begin to notice these changes during the menopausal years. A dry vagina can lead to discomfort and perhaps pain during love making. Lower estrogen levels mean there is less protective natural lubrication on the vaginal tissue, and some women therefore are more vulnerable to vaginal infection.

"I had vaginal dryness, but I have K-Y jelly; it's very good." (*Brenda*)

"I've had a lot of vaginal itching; I had a terrible time for about three years. I used all sorts of creams. Nothing seemed to work for very long. I stopped wearing tights because of it." (*Rosie*)

"The only real symptom after the menopause was dryness of the vagina, which meant that I was rather prone to infections." (*Geraldine*)

"I didn't like the increase in vaginal dryness that came. But obviously one can cope with that and I do." (*Angela*)

Nearly half of our interviewees noticed this symptom. We'll look at ways of dealing with it in Chapter 7.

Bladder Problems

Although the bladder is not technically part of the genitals, changes at the menopause can also involve the bladder because of its proximity to the uterus and the vagina.

The membrane of the bladder, like the membrane of the vagina, can become thinner, and this may lead to increased frequency of passing urine, together with a greater feeling of urgency.

None of the 15 women we interviewed mentioned any symptoms specifically concerning the bladder.

Insomnia and Tiredness

This is another symptom associated with the menopause, but there is little evidence that it is directly related. Five of our interviewees mentioned insomnia and a changing sleep pattern as part of their experience, but this was often a consequence of either waking up in the middle of a sweat and having to change the bedclothes, or needing to urinate in the middle of the night. Inevitably, if your sleep pattern is interrupted, you'll be more tired. Four of our interviewees reported this as a serious symptom. Two related it to broken sleep, one to getting older, and the fourth to the demands and stress of moving house at that particular time in her life.

Formication (Crawling Sensation)

The term "formication" is derived from the Latin word for ant; it's very apt because this experience can feel exactly as if insects are crawling all over your skin.

"I thought I had a mite under the skin. It was terrible; I kept scratching." (*Maureen*)

"I had this feeling that things were running all over me. I remember sitting in class thinking, 'What on earth is happening to me?'" (*Geraldine*)

Three of our interviewees experienced this sensation after their last menstrual period. No one seems to know what causes it; nevertheless, it is accepted as a symptom of the menopause.

Skin Changes

Skin change in our genitals is directly related to the lowering production of estrogen by our ovaries. But because of a combination of the aging process and the fall of the estrogen level, the skin on the rest of our body changes as well. Very nearly all our interviewees had noticed their skin changing:

"I can see dryness and the beginnings of the loss of elasticity." (*Bea*)

"My skin felt as if it were drawn tight. It was very dry and I couldn't put enough stuff on it. I got eczema around the base of my neck and odd patches on both hands. Sometimes under my arms tremendous itchy patches, and my scalp itched like mad." (*Anne*)

"I was just starting to be menopausal. I got this terrible irritation. I got eczema, believe it or not, on the bottom of one of my feet." (*Sheila*)

The membrane of the nostrils, like the membrane of the vagina, can lose moisture.

"My skin has become dry and I have irritation spots like in my elbows – in fact on all sweat points – and I noticed that the interior of my nose was very dry and irritated." (*Doreen*)

"A funny thing I've noticed on my face, I've got a little dark mark there, which I've only noticed in the last three years." (*Brenda*)

The most obvious signs of changes are dryness, increasing wrinkles as the elasticity is lost, and dark spots on the skin, especially on the backs of the hands. It is mainly white women whose skin alters in these ways – especially in the areas of the skin exposed to the light. Women with black or brown skin escape these changes because the melanin, or pigmentation, in their skin protects it from the effect of ultraviolet light.

Aching Joints and Muscles

With lower levels of estrogen, muscle strength is reduced. Nearly half the women interviewed experienced aches and pains during the menopausal years. Maureen said: "My knees conked out. I stopped working because I just couldn't walk." Angela found that her "legs ached a lot and walking was difficult." "I had pains in my elbows and knees," said Rose, "and especially my shoulders."

Strictly speaking, the symptoms regarded as *directly* related to menopause – physical events that can cause mild or severe distress – are hot flushes, night sweats, and vaginal dryness. Other symptoms are more easily attributed to the aging process in general, because our muscles and skin tissue change as we get older, and so do our bones.

Our Bones and Osteoporosis

After the menopause, bones lose their density and become porous. If you imagine the difference between a piece of foam rubber and a piece of natural sponge, you will get an idea of the difference between a dense bone and a porous bone. The more porous – that is, the more holes – the more brittle the bone will be. Before menopause, estrogen helps to retain calcium from our food, which is used by our bodies to maintain our bones. After the menopause, with diminished estrogen, we retain calcium less easily. This means that without due care and attention, our bones become more porous and more brittle, possibly resulting in osteoporosis, or brittle-bone disease.

This disease is associated with elderly women, who very easily fracture a hip bone or wrist bone, or twist the spine in a fall, and the consequences are very serious. Bones in both men and women begin to lose density at about the age of thirty, but after the menopause, this occurs at an accelerated rate. One in every four women is said to be vulnerable to osteoporosis in later life, but nobody as yet knows how to predict precisely which 25 percent of women will be at risk.

One thing we do know: osteoporosis is rare among black people, whereas both Asian and Caucasian people are more prone to it. This suggests that some people have denser bones than others to start with. Research also shows that bone density can be affected positively by diet and exercise, especially if this is attended to earlier in our lives.

"How dense we've managed to get our bones by the time we approach our mid-thirties is the key factor to how we'll stand up to the increased bone loss after menopause. If a woman hasn't eaten properly and hasn't taken the right sort of exercise, then her bone system is already pretty light, so it only takes that bit of increased bone loss after menopause to make it appear the menopause has caused the osteoporosis. Women with denser, heavier bones and who've been educated to look after themselves have much more chance." (*Jo*)

"If you have a woman who doesn't exercise, who's Caucasian rather than Negroid, who has a calcium-deficient diet, the consequences in terms of osteoporosis will be greater for her than for someone who is the opposite." (*Siddle*)

We explore the subject of osteoporosis further in Chapter 7; because this disease is currently receiving a lot of publicity. But now, having reviewed the major physical characteristics of the menopause, we look at some of the possible emotional repercussions.

4

Going Crazy?

———

IT'S not surprising that with so many physiological changes at this time, we may notice that our thoughts, attitudes, and feelings also seem to be affected. Our perceptions of ourselves and others in our lives can alter.

A wide category of experiences reported by the women we interviewed can be loosely termed "psychological." But before we look at these particular experiences, it's important to state that no actual psychological disorder is associated with the menopause. Some of the myths about "mad menopausal women" probably stem from a clinical disorder labeled "involutional melancholia," otherwise known as menopausal depression. How it came to be classified as a mental disorder in the past we can only surmise. But many studies carried out in the past twenty years to find evidence linking depression directly to the menopause have failed to detect any.

However, having said that there is no clinical reason for depression, we don't mean that you may not feel depressed at this time.

Any of the psychological symptoms described here is a combination of hormonal changes, social and environmental factors, and of course the aging process in general. All of these can contribute some kind of stress.

"Stopping your periods, hot flushes, night sweats, and a dry vagina are the only symptoms that can be shown to be directly related to estrogen withdrawal. All the other things are related to midlife transition, or crisis, or to premenstrual tension that would classically change with the menstrual cycle." (*Last*)

"When I say depression I mean a global loss of function, loss of energy, loss of interest in life: 'I don't want to go out, my memory has gone, I've lost my sparkle, the world is gray and flat.' It's not depression, it's a depressed mood." (*Siddle*)

Most women find their emotions difficult to understand and manage at the best of times. We tend to be frightened of our feelings because they are irrational, and we can't always explain why we feel a particular way. We're frightened of our feelings because they appear to be overwhelming and powerful, and under their influence we behave in ways we label as childish, uncontrollable, or socially unacceptable.

In truth, our feelings do not exist as separate entities outside our bodies. Feelings are influenced by physical factors, and at any time of physical change, we are quite likely to experience some kind of emotional turmoil. Although nothing inevitably connects the menopause to depression or anxiety, several of the women we interviewed felt the emotional aspect had been, or was still, an important part of their experience.

"I just knew all day I was crying inside; nobody else knew. As I walked across the street I used to think, 'I can't do it. I'll never get across the road. I'm going to have to ask someone to take me.' I didn't want to go to the school gates, where I'd have to speak to people. I didn't want anything to do with people, which was quite alien to everything I'd always been. I felt I became a different person; I didn't recognize myself during that six months." (*Diana*)

"I'd feel very depressed for no reason. And sometimes very angry. I would flare up at the least little thing; I'd just blow my top." (*Rosie*).

"I was in a completely childish panic. It's the sense of being out of control that is very distinct." (*Anne*)

"I think there's a feeling of being over the hill. Being useless now, somehow you're not really worth anything." (*Geraldine*)

"My shoulders ached and that's exactly how I felt. I used to walk around thinking, 'This is my role in life—to be a burden.'" (*Diana*)

"Apart from a long period of depression I remember short bits of plummeting. At some point I remember thinking that this was like PMT (premenstrual tension) but for about three years. I felt very out of touch with my body: that I didn't know it, I didn't understand what it was going to do. I was very disoriented—like the early stages of pregnancy, but when you're pregnant it's in aid of something. It also felt very like adolescence, when lots of things are happening to your body and you don't understand the changes and you're becoming something different. But then you're expecting something nice at the end. Now there's just a question mark." (*Angela*)

"Sometimes I felt depressed with it, but not the sort that are right down in the depths that some people do." (*Brenda*)

"I can remember praying 'Why have you brought me to this state? I was happy as I was.'" (*Diana*)

"At first I could still cope with everyday living and then suddenly it seemed to happen. I couldn't cope any more, with the tiredness and the depression, and this in itself was frightening because I didn't know why I was feeling like this." (*Rosie*)

"I realized that understanding it makes an enormous difference, and other people accepting it. Because otherwise you feel you're going mad. Feeling mad is sort of protest, you know: 'Can't anybody see what's going on here; I'll end up in the loony bin if you don't look after me.' It really does feel like that." (*Angela*)

"Part of this vulnerability is connected with increased anxiety; it's a fragility that links it all." (*Bea*)

Experiencing swings of mood and difficult emotions isn't in itself negative. We can often learn from our feelings if we accept them. But because of the cultural taboo on talking openly about feelings—let alone expressing them during this time—women can fall into the trap of trying to bottle up and control their feelings excessively, instead of acknowledging them, talking about them, and trusting them.

Stress

Although many women pass through this time without noticing any change, the majority of us are likely to feel something. If there is a noticeable cyclic pattern to moods, it may well be associated with hormonal change. But this may just be premenstrual tension—not necessarily a symptom of the menopause.

The sense of being out of control is commonly described because there is no distinct pattern of menopausal change. Living with unpredictability can be stressful. There can be a feeling of sadness as the reproductive cycle comes to an end; even if a woman does not actually want to have more children, she can be aware of the ending of a major part of her life. For a woman who has not had children and has wanted to, this can be a time of realization that there is a point at which she cannot go on hoping.

"It takes some time dawning, but it's a tremendously difficult time for infertile women, who've never been pregnant because they at long last realize they must come to terms with the problem that they're *never* going to have children. So they begin to look at life with a different perspective." (*McGarry*)

This can also apply to women who are not necessarily infertile but who, for many different reasons, have postponed having children and now find that it's no longer an option.

We also feel angry toward our bodies. This sounds irrational, but it is very easy to get frustrated when this body we have known fairly well acts unpredictably and also appears to be letting us down. We may be worried about getting older and anxious about losing our attractiveness, either in general or to a sexual partner.

Another source of stress comes from whatever else is happening in our lives around this time. It's well known that menopause in a woman's life often coincides with children leaving home and her parents getting ill or dying.

During her menopause Diana moved house to a different part of the country and was going through a difficult time with her husband. Anne changed her job and took on a very demanding workload. Geraldine's husband started having an affair with a younger woman: "For a whole year he was having an affair and I was setting up this health education unit, and the person in charge was a difficult woman so there was a lot of stress that year."

Sometimes stress symptoms can be wrongly labeled menopausal. Hot and cold flushes, palpitations, or anxiety attacks can be experienced by both young men and women and by middle-aged men in stressful situations. As one of the people we interviewed remarked: "The menopause is sometimes a convenient tag on which to hang any emotional or so-called irrational behavior."

"It's a bit like when a baby is teething, isn't it? When women get to that age, everything is blamed on the menopause. I think you ought to be aware that not everything you suffer is menopausal, and there's a danger that it's just dismissed as being menopausal, when there could be something underlying it." (*Sheila*)

Emotional outbursts, depression, and irritability can be triggered by external factors alone:

"One woman came in last week at forty-three having been told she was menopausal. What she's got is a twenty-year-old mentally-retarded son, looked after at home; a four-year-old daughter; and a seventeen-year-old son taking his exams; and although her husband is very caring, he goes out at 7:30 in the morning and comes back at 8:00 at night. It's just too much but it's not the menopause." (*Last*)

Our reactions to the menopause have to be understood as a complex interweaving of all these factors to a greater or lesser extent. "That's what makes it so interesting," said Julie Endacott, "but so difficult pinpointing what are purely physical symptoms due to deficiencies and which are additive symptoms due to other problems that surround a woman at this time."

5

Sex and Sexuality

WHEN we look at how our sexuality can be affected by the changes occurring during menopause, it's important to separate the changes associated with the menopause itself from the longer-term changes that occur very gradually, over a period of time, as a result of getting older.

Research shows that the level of sexual interest starts to fall and continues to decline in both men and women in middle age. When researchers measure sexual interest, they usually base their measurement on the frequency of sexual activity and the kind of activity – in other words, what you do and how often you do it! And the normal point of measurement is sexual intercourse, which is dependent on the man's ability to obtain and maintain an erection. Measuring sexual arousal in women is much more complex because there's no such obvious point of measurement.

In order to see how female arousal can be affected by the menopause, we need to look at what affects our sexual arousal at any other times in our lives.

Arousal is an umbrella term that describes a pattern of changes affecting body and mind simultaneously. Sexual arousal is triggered by a stimulus – a thought, a touch, a word, a picture – that prompts the brain to set in motion various responses, including an increase of the blood flow into the abdominal and pelvic area. If you're relaxed, your level of arousal will increase as the pleasurable stimulus increases. Your body will follow a cycle, arousal increasing with pleasure, until you reach a peak of some kind, when you may experience a release.

In order to become absorbed in our physical sensations, we need to become less aware of what's going on outside our bodies and temporarily more aware of the sensations *inside* our bodies. This is why, when sexually aroused, we can be temporarily oblivious of minor physical discomfort, such as cold, hunger, or a cramped position. But as soon as the arousal dissipates we become acutely aware again of our surroundings and situation.

Lack of interest in sex and sexual difficulties generally can often be traced to insufficient arousal. Although many women tend to depend on their partners to provide them with sexual stimulation and satisfaction, the key to arousal lies in *ourselves*.

Several factors make it difficult or even impossible for us to get sexually excited: for example, tiredness, recent surgery, nausea, the effect of alcohol, and various kinds of medication, including antidepressants and tranquilizers. Another major physical factor is any kind of pain, tenderness, or discomfort.

One of the commonest causes of difficulties with sex at the menopause is a dry vagina. A woman may feel eager to make love and then find that intercourse is painful, because her vagina is dry and the tissue not as yielding as before. We've already described how this is directly related to lowering estrogen levels, although it's important to remember that lack of lubrication is not something that only menopausal women suffer from. It can happen at any age, to any woman.

A frequently prescribed remedy for vaginal dryness is K-Y jelly. Another remedy, particularly helpful during menopause, is estrogen cream, which not only increases the amount of estrogen acting locally on the vaginal wall but is also absorbed into the bloodstream. The combined local and systemic effect is to thicken the tissues of the vagina, which in turn produce more mucus so that the vagina becomes properly lubricated.

One of the biggest passion-killers of all, however, is *anxiety*. Worry of any kind can interfere with the process of sexual arousal. This may be something quite unconnected with sex—for example, problems with people at home or at work—or may be related specifically to sex itself, like fear of discomfort and pain. This is why one painful experience can set up a negative cycle because we then anticipate discomfort, and the anxiety keeps us from becoming aroused and naturally lubricated, which in turn leads to more discomfort, and so it goes on.

While vaginal dryness is frequently highlighted as a negative aspect of the menopause, there is also a great positive aspect for many women. Fear of pregnancy can strongly inhibit our ability to let go and become sexually aroused, not only perhaps because of some distaste at having to use the paraphernalia associated with contraception, but also because of a deep-seated fear as to whether it really will be safe. Many women undoubtedly therefore experience great relief after the menopause because of a new sense of freedom.

If liberation from contraception is an obvious positive factor in a woman's enjoyment of sex with male partners, it can also be a relief for some of the men.

"He's just terribly relieved because he's always felt bad, always felt guilty. And he's been saying for years he ought to go and get a vasectomy." (*Sylvia*)

According to a survey carried out in 1983, 40 percent of women over forty in sexually active relationships no longer ran the risk of pregnancy because either the woman or her partner had been sterilized.

If you are in a sexually active relationship and have not been sterilized by either specific sterilization surgery, such as tubular ligation (typing of both fallopian tubes to prevent fertilization of the eggs), or hysterectomy, or your partner has not had a vasectomy, then contraception will still be a concern.

When Can I Stop Using Contraception?

When can you be sure that contraception is no longer necessary? When do we cease to be fertile?

The answer depends on how long each one of us continues to

ovulate. As long as the egg is released the possibility of conception exists, which is why even during the erratic cycles of the menopause, a woman in her early fifties can become pregnant.

Many women judge the situation for themselves and stop using contraception without asking advice, but check it out later. Doctors' advice varies. Sylvia experienced an earlier-than-usual menopause at forty-one and was told by her physician, when she asked for her coil to be removed, that she should keep it in for two years after her last period. Angela at fifty-plus was also told to use contraception for at least two years after her last period. But she found it problematic because she was never quite sure whether the last period she'd had was in fact the final one.

Even though we can have periods, it is unlikely that we will ovulate with that period. The accepted rule is that the *majority* of women are not fertile after fifty years of age. "I think you should continue to use some method of contraception for one year before fifty and six months after fifty. If you haven't had a period for six months after fifty, you'd be very, very unlikely to conceive. Even though you can have a period after that time, the chances of your ovulating with that period must be fairly zilch. But it is terribly difficult to be absolutely sure that you're safe." (*Last*)

The golden rule seems to be if you begin the menopause before fifty, then you should continue with contraception for two years following your last menstruation. If you begin the menopause after fifty, then you should continue with contraception for one year following your last period.

Contraceptive Choice

The choice of contraceptive method is usually one of the mechanical methods—a condom, spermicidal foams, or creams and suppositories in conjunction with a diaphragm—or an intrauterine contraceptive device (IUD). For the women who use an IUD or coil, it is vital to remember the following caution: "Irregular bleeding must never be ascribed to the IUD. You can't say that because you've got a coil in, that's why you're having spotting. If you've got regular periods with an IUD that's fine, but if you're starting to spot or get quite a regular loss, then it should be carefully investigated." (*Last*)

The Pill

About 5 percent of women use the contraceptive pill in their late forties. Contraceptive pills are composed of varying balances of the hormones estrogen and progestogen, which are taken together or separately.

Because of risk of thrombosis associated with estrogen, the estrogen/progestogen combination pills are not recommended for women even in perfect health over the age of forty, or for women, if they smoke, over thirty-five. However comfortable a woman has felt on a combination pill, she will be strongly advised to stop taking it as she approaches middle age.

On the other hand, the progestogen-only pill (the minipill, as it is sometimes called) is frequently prescribed at this time. One of the side effects of the additional progestogen is that it suppresses FSH (see Chapter 1), which helps prevent flushing. This can be seen as a specific advantage, but the disadvantages are that it suppresses menstruation (amenorrhea), which will affect the pattern of bleeding. A danger in this instance is for women to let this unusual pattern continue, believing it to be quite a normal occurrence, because irregular blood loss *can* be indicative of some abnormality such as polyps or endometrial cancer. For this reason it is *essential* to report any irregular bleeding so that it can be investigated immediately. Other checks, such as blood pressure, will have to be maintained as well if you are taking this pill.

Injectables

Progestogen is sometimes administered as a hormonal contraceptive in an injectable form. A woman is injected with the contraceptive every three months. This would be advisable only for women *already using* this method before menopause. The side effects and dangers are the same as with the progestogen oral contraceptive.

IUD (Intrauterine Device)

This method of contraception works by inhibiting implantation of the fertilized ovum. It does not interfere with the body's normal hormone activity. Because an IUD should not cause irregular bleeding, any menstrual irregularity experienced by a woman with IUD should be immediately investigated. IUDs are now used with caution because of the risks of side effects or injury.

Diaphragm

This is a recommended form of contraception during the menopause because it is safe and because the jelly or spermicidal cream also helps to act as a lubricant if a woman's vagina is dry.

The trouble is that many women find them clumsy and inhibiting to sexual pleasure. Protection is similar if the cervical cap is used, and this has the advantage over the diaphragm in that it can be left in place.

Sheath/Condom

Recommended, but some men find them a turnoff. However, they have recently become more generally accepted because of the spread of AIDS.

Spermicides

Spermicidal potions come in all sorts of forms: creams, jellies, foams, tablets, and suppositories.

The Rhythm Method

We haven't included the rhythm method because it is the most unreliable form of contraception during the menopause. A woman's cycles are often anovulatory at the end of her reproductive life, as they were at the beginning, and it is extremely difficult to know when your cycle is ovulatory during the menopause and when it isn't. Since the rhythm method relies on certainty of the time of ovulation, it is not recommended.

Changing Attitudes

While looking at the benefits of this new-found freedom a woman has to take into account her sexual motivation and whether or not she's still attracted to her sexual partner. "She may have gone off him, which a lot of women won't accept themselves. They don't actually like him; they don't want him; but they say, "It's the menopause." (*Last*)

Cooling off toward a partner can simply be a temporary state, which most people experience at some time or another in relationships. We can feel angry, resentful, or hurt by what a partner has done or said at some time, and it is easy for unexpressed feelings to find their way into the bedroom, forming an unseen obstacle to feeling open enough to want to make love.

On the other hand, it may be more permanent; and if a relationship is no longer sexual, then a woman will have to make her own choice as to whether to stay in that relationship because she loves her partner even though there is no sexual interaction, or to leave the relationship if there is no fulfillment at any level at all.

Our interviewees noted a variety of changes:

"I think if anything I'd say "more fluctuation." Sometimes I can feel surprisingly more erotic or more sexually aroused, sort of more intense about it, and another time I won't be quite so interested. I might have felt that before, but somehow there's an intensity at both ends." (*Bea*)

"I feel sometimes that I ought to be having intercourse more often for his sake, but he doesn't seem to be worried, and if he feels like it you know I'm always quite happy, but I don't get these intense feelings anymore." (*Sheila*)

"I'm learning to enjoy myself and enjoy my body and feel good about my sexuality again, having finally after all these years shipped off the 'sexy lady of the 50s' image which has been a bitch to get rid of, it's so ingrained." (*Jo*)

"I think having an affair in my early fifties was marvelous for me and I felt waked up in a way that I hadn't, which was really sad, I think. But I felt wonderful, and so it may have been the beginning of my accepting my body, and so sex or not, I feel much happier." (*Geraldine*)

"I probably feel more sexual, actually, because I was feeling liberated and because of the need for contact, and that's a wonderful feeling." (*Angela*)

Sexuality at the Menopause

Our sexuality is greatly affected by our attitudes and expectations. First, there is a myth in our society that after menopause, women are "past it." This stems from the association of sexual activity with reproductive ability alone; once fertility is over, sex is thought to be irrelevant.

It's true that if a woman has only endured sex because she wanted to conceive, then after menopause there is a sense that is is not worth it any more. "When they've done what they've set out to do, they no longer want the hassle of it all." (*Last*)

Although in recent years the women's movement has encouraged women not to believe that this is necessarily so, the bulk of medical opinion still insists that declining estrogen will have an adverse effect on a woman's sexual response. That it does have an effect is true, but no one can say how significant an effect it will be. The hormonal change is only one of many factors, and its effect has to be considered in relation to everything else.

There is, for example, hormonal evidence to show that women's sexual desire (libido) is related to the level of testosterone produced; so one might anticipate that with more testosterone being converted into estrogen at this time, perhaps the libido will lessen. However, if a woman at this time is enjoying the liberation of sex without contraception and she is able to experience more arousal as a result, then who is to say which factor is going to have more effect?

It is clear that of all the factors that influence our sexuality at this time, the specific influence of hormonal change is not all-important. Although estrogen replacement therapy can help particularly severe menopausal symptoms, it would be wrong to believe that a woman can enjoy sex after the menopause only if her genitals are restored to their pristine premenopausal condition. This is little short of saying that sex is still only for the young and that if you're on the "wrong" side of fifty, you have to rejuvenate your body in order to be sexual.

Another important factor affecting our sexuality is dependence on a mate. This implies the need to continue to appear sexually attractive in a society that favors youth, smooth skin, and slimness over middle age, wrinkles and spare tires. However confident a woman feels in other areas of her life, she may find herself worrying about losing her attractiveness to a particular partner and consequently feeling more desperate about his still finding her desirable.

Misunderstanding can easily occur if the man in question is at a similar age and therefore experiencing his own sexual changes. He may well find himself less able to act on his sexual interest – in other words, not able to get an erection so easily. The woman in these circumstances may easily interpret this as proof that she is losing her appeal, and feel rejected without realizing that it has more to do with *him* and how *he* feels. This same insecurity can lead us simply to dismiss ourselves as unattractive, and to take ourselves out of the running. As Anne put it, "I felt some time ago that I was out of the mating game, but it didn't matter."

Angela felt that the reality was in favor of younger women.

"However much you say, 'Older women are maturer and sexually they're more mature, and so on . . . nevertheless, put yourself and a young woman in front of a man; of course he'll go for the young one because you yourself feel, when you look at younger people, that yes, they have something that you appreciate that you're sad to be leaving."

Angela consciously looked for women who were high-powered and starting out on a new career after fifty, as role models, but found that the possibility of beauty after this age gave her much more encouragement:

"*Harpers & Queen* at one point had an over-fifties edition, which I absolutely rushed for. I wanted to see all these beautiful women, like Sophia Loren and the rest of them, really looking handsome. I've got a suspicion that did more for me than the image of the woman making a success of her career!"

It is difficult to avoid cultural pressure to be young and beautiful and, more importantly, one of a couple.

However, it's important to remember that not all women are in relationships; not all women are in relationships with men; and not all women who are in relationships with men want intercourse to be the only means of giving and receiving.

Options

Heterosexual intercourse is not the only choice open to women as a means of continuing sexual activity after the menopause. There are alternatives.

Self-Pleasuring

The unfortunate thing about masturbation is the word itself, which doesn't give any indication of the kind of experience it can be. Masturbation has long been, and still is, forbidden by various religions. Even from a secular point of view, it's considered a fourth-rate activity: a little sordid, usually indulged in by young boys or old men, and a rather self-degrading activity.

But many women do masturbate. Some masturbate as an extension of their sexual activity with their partners, and some when they are alone, as physical release or specific sexual release, or sometimes as a way of self-loving and enjoying their bodies.

Self-stimulation with your finger, a vibrator, or running water, or rubbing yourself against something can be pleasurable and lead to orgasm. The sexual arousal experienced both psychologically and physiologically can be very satisfying: neither more satisfying nor less satisfying than with a partner—just different. If you want a "good" reason for doing it, this kind of self-stimulation certainly helps to keep the vagina in a healthy condition!

Other Sexual Pleasures

Heterosexual sex is not the only way to keep sexually active. Women who choose other women as sexual partners experience menopause in the same way, and sexual activity between them is subject to the same ups and downs. But continuing sexual stimulus can play just as important and beneficial a part as with a heterosexual couple.

We must remember, too, that there are many sexual activities you can enjoy together apart from intercourse, which many heterosexual couples enjoy for all sorts of different reasons. Oral sex and mutual stimulation are just two alternatives. It may well be that reducing the emphasis on intercourse could enhance sexual pleasure for many women, not to mention their partners.

If you have always had an enjoyable sexual relationship with a partner, then it's quite likely you will continue through and after the menopause and be able to accommodate any specific changes that may occur. As ever, the key is clear and caring communication.

6

Seeking Help

MANY women pass through menopause without noticing anything untoward, as we have said earlier. An even greater number do notice physical changes in their bodies but are not unduly distressed by them. However, there are times when women seek help either because of the severity of the symptoms or because of the length of time these symptoms continue.

It's important to maintain a balance between the two prevalent attitudes towards the menopause—between the view that the menopause is a clinical syndrome or an illness for which one must be treated, and the "no backbone" view, which claims that only a spineless woman can't cope and that she should endeavor to put mind over matter. "I think attitudes help enormously. It's not to say that a woman only gets symptoms because she's got a negative attitude, because that's not true, and I think they're made to feel guilty if they do then get symptoms." (*Last*)

The first person a woman is likely to seek help from is her physician. The successful outcome of this step will depend very much on the knowledge and attitude of the particular physician, not only to menopausal symptoms but also to the risks attached to the various kinds of treatment available.

Some of the women we interviewed reported varying, and in several cases unsatisfactory, experiences:

"I had an old-fashioned doctor who said, 'Either it will get better or it won't.' This irritated me because I didn't seek advice lightly, so when I did go, I wanted something more positive. I only went when I was really desperately thinking there must be something wrong with me. But he was in his sixties." (*Diana*)

Eventually Diana asked for treatment and went to her local family planning clinic, where she was prescribed a contraceptive pill.

"My physician was a woman who was actually at school with me. She was helpful as much as she could be; we just talked over things to see what I'd like to do. She asked if I wanted HRT (hormone replacement therapy) and I said 'Absolutely no.'" (*Angela*)

"I just felt for my own comfort I'd go and discuss it with a doctor. He was very dubious about recommending anything, and said 'I could give you these to help, but they do have side effects and they're not very nice'—so that's about as much as I got from him." (*Doreen*)

"I went to my own physician and told him that I'd flush just when dropping off to sleep at night and I'd sweat and it would wake me up. He said, 'It's probably postural. Does it happen when you lie down during the day?' Really, can you imagine how often I lie down during the day! A real lack of insight—'It's postural, so get on with it!' He's a young physician and usually pretty good, and I was quite surprised." (*Sheila*)

"I would be at the doctor's every couple of weeks. But I couldn't tell him what was wrong with me. He'd say, 'Hello, Rosie, what can I do for you?' and I'd just sit there and burst into tears." (*Rosie*)

"I think a lot of physicians recognize the problem but decide that they don't want to deal with it. They either don't have the time, or don't know what they're doing, or they'd rather you'd follow it up at the hospital." (*Butler*)

We might go to our physician for reassurance, information about what's going on and prescription for something that will help, or a referral to a specialist—either a consultant gynecologist or an alternative health practitioner.

Types of Problems Needing Help

What are the usual symptoms for which women seek specialist help?

"The majority of women come to the clinic with hot flushes, insomnia, palpitations, and, very frequently, night sweats. Another group has vaginal problems, dryness, or pain on intercourse; loss of libido is very common as well. And then there's the third group with psychological problems, depression, loss of confidence, lack of concentration." (*Endacott*) "Complaints by their menfolk, feelings of inadequacy, feelings that they want to take sensible health precautions, or wanting HRT to promote a healthy old age." (*Last*)

What Happens With a Specialist?

If you do seek the help of a specialist, what can you expect?

"The first thing is to make the diagnosis; the second is 'OK, so you have those problems, but why did you come to see me? Was it for information, or do you want something done? If so, which symptoms trouble you the most, and how much?' The third thing is 'Do you have any medical problems or difficulties that you need to talk about?' Essentially, we're doing a health screen. You're offering absolutely super-duper general practice, really. You're talking about health and wellbeing and you bring in all sorts of other information about major life events which have occurred and could be troubling you." (*Siddle*)

Diagnosis

In some cases it's obvious that if your last period is over and you are of a certain age, you are describing a postmenopausal condition. But if the specialist needs to be sure, a hormone test is carried out.

This can be a smear test which involves measuring the cell growth in the vagina to indicate the level of estrogen in your body. Unfortunately, a smear test is not an absolutely reliable indication as to whether or not a woman is menopausal. Other factors such as time of cycle, use of other medication, recent intercourse, and vaginal infection also affect the cell growth in the vagina.

Another method of hormonal measurement is a blood test. This measures the level of FSH (follicle stimulating hormone; see Chapter 1). If you stop ovulating, the FSH remains very high. But again, this method is not foolproof in diagnosing the menopause, for the following reasons: "It depends on the stage in your cycle, what level you're going to find. If it's at the beginning of your cycle you'll find high levels of FSH anyway. There's a great deal of overlap between what is menopausal and what's a normal cycle. Also, when you're taking a blood test, you're taking it in one moment of time. A better way to do it is testing urine and do a 24-hour measurement of the excretory products of estrogen in the urine. Then you can tell how much you are making. But that's tedious and it means carrying big bottles around, so people don't do it." (*Last*)

This gynecologist cautioned against a misdiagnosis resulting in hormone replacement therapy (HRT) being given too early. "If at forty-eight a woman is almost menopausal, maybe she's not going to have menopause until she's fifty-two. If she takes HRT it'll suppress her normal production of hormones anyway. I've had several patients who've been put on HRT too soon." (*Last*)

Fortunately, when Geraldine took herself to a specialist in her late forties, her experience was positive.

"It was so strange to be treated nicely and intelligently and also for people to have accurate information because they took tests and I was told that I had a high estrogen level, that I was fit, and my vaginal walls were in good shape, to get on with life, as I hadn't got the menopause yet, and so I felt, oh, fine."

Treatments

Diagnosis is followed by a discussion between a woman and her specialist about her symptoms, their severity, and the possibilities of treatment.

"I would like a woman to come into my office and say, 'The

symptoms I have sound as if I'm menopausal. I've read about the menopause; I know what causes it. I know what the symptoms are. I know what the consequences of long-term estrogen treatment are. I feel that my symptoms are sufficient to warrant my trying some treatment. I'd like to try it to see if it makes me feel better, and I'd like to be able to talk to you as we go along about how long I continue with my treatment.'" (*Siddle*)

This portrait of an ideal patient does presuppose quite a lot of information, fluency, and confidence on the part of the woman concerned, but it shows that some specialists are willing to look at treatment as a cooperative venture. Certainly, if a woman has the information, she is in a much better position to make the appropriate choices. Nicholas Siddle emphasized the need for more general education:

"When one is involved in the menopause, one thing is quite self-evident. Five percent of the time is spent on medical matters and diagnosis; the health screening, which is a useful part of the follow-up, takes up 25 percent; a further 15 percent is taken up on minor adjustments to treatment to fit the individual; 50 percent of the time and benefit is the value of having someone to talk to. That's why there would be an enormous benefit in more family planning clinics and well woman clinics taking on an educational role. A counseling facility for women in this situation must be pressed for, even politicized if you like; it has to be promoted because the general practitioner can't possibly cope. There aren't sufficient clinics of a medical nature to achieve that for women, so it's got to be provided by lay-type organizations. Better education would be enormously helpful. I believe that some women can certainly be helped to deal with the distress that is caused by the menopause, without necessarily any recourse to treatment."

Before an agreement on treatment is reached, an extensive medical history must be taken, and a physical examination completed, in order to eliminate the known risk factors associated with estrogen therapy (see Chapter 7).

Also, as we mentioned earlier, any treatment must be accompanied by regular supervision.

Menopause Groups

We talked to two women, Jo and Rosie, who run self-help discussion groups for women in the menopause. Jo runs courses in a local community education context.

"Some people come because they want to learn more about the menopause; others because they're depressed. The most common statement that comes up is 'I feel I'm at a crossroads in life.' It's becoming more remarkable the longer I run courses, just how many women are saying they feel something wrong and they don't know what it is they want."

Rosie was recommended to her group by her physician, whose nurse was running the group at the time. They met once a month, and she went for two years. Having gotten so much out of it, Rosie took the group over when the nurse left.

"I learned so much. It related to how I was feeling and what was happening to me. I felt so much better when I came out. It was the women themselves talking that was reassuring. I realized I wasn't going out of my mind. Each session I learned something new, and I heard the women talk about things that happened to them. I knew that if I did experience those things, I wouldn't need to go running to the doctor because I knew it was all part of the menopause. Although I'd still have days when I was really down, when I would scream and shout at my husband, I knew now what was causing it. I was able to tell him why I was like this."

One of the difficulties both women acknowledged is that women find it difficult to come to a group of this kind at first. Jo felt it was because they didn't want to make a statement about why they were leaving the house. "Many women can't actually say, 'Get your own supper tonight; I'm going to evening school.' A lot of them don't even say what the class is. There's a lot of hostility from families because it's not like going to a crafts course. It's considered to be self-indulgent, going off to gossip, and not necessary in some way." Rosie said, "During the menopause it's too much of an effort to get up and go just when you need it most, so it's very difficult to get people to come along."

The main benefit of attending a group is removal of the sense of isolation:

"I think a lot of it is just being able to speak to someone that's been through it, or is going through and has been through the same thing. It's the same old story of realizing that you're not the only one." (*Butler*)

We may need to set up this formal structure for talking because our culture does not allow for this kind of exchange of experience in the natural course of daily life. It's interesting to see how this can occur, for example, in Sri Lanka:

"In many rural areas of developing countries, women spend six to seven hours doing household chores that take less than one hour in developed places. Here you turn on a tap and you get your water; cooking is done using gas or electricity, which is available again at the end of a switch. If you have to go to fetch your water or collect firewood, this involves very often long journeys, sometimes up to three or four miles. Usually women go together in little groups. During the journey they talk to each other. By this means they get the social interaction and also the kind of cushioning from problems associated with life changes such as menopause. I think this does help resolve some of the stress problems associated with menopause." (*Senanayake*)

We are often more isolated from each other in this culture, and we came across only a few groups in our research. However, we have heard that more women are taking the initiative in setting up groups or classes, so if you're interested it may be worth checking with your physician or local family planning clinic to see if there is a group in your area.

7

Treatment

IF you seek help from your physician, you'll probably be offered hormone replacement therapy (HRT) because it is considered the only fast and effective treatment for flushes, sweating, and vaginal dryness.

Hormone Replacement Therapy

HRT describes the introduction of extra hormones into the bloodstream to replace our own estrogen supplies, which are waning naturally as a result of the gradual ovarian function decline. Although the name suggests that this medication simply replaces your normal hormones with the same substances, it is a little misleading.

First, the so-called "natural" estrogens used are not natural in the sense that they do not normally occur in humans. They are manufactured estrogens, *similar* to the body's own, but with different effects. Sometimes estrogen is derived from the urine of pregnant mares, because their urine contains a highly powerful estrogen; but again, this cannot be considered truly natural to humans, although it is to horses.

As the ovary fails we lose *estradiol*, the major estrogen compound. Estradiol cannot be manufactured outside the body, so it is *estrone*, one of the weaker estrogen compounds, that is administered in hormone replacement therapy.

Second, however advanced the research and technology in manufacturing these compounds may be, they can never match the body's own delicate mechanism, which maintains the amount of estrogen in the blood at the correct level. And finally, since estrogens are broken down and cleared from the bloodstream quickly, very high levels have to be given in order to maintain an adequate level for twenty-four hours each day to relieve both symptoms – hot flushes in the daytime and sweating at night. As you can see, HRT is not true hormone replacement therapy; more correctly, it's the best that can be done in the circumstances.

The History of HRT

Estrogen therapy has been around for almost half a century. It was commonly used in the past in the treatment of menopausal symptoms in women, much more widely in the United States than in the United Kingdom. HRT was popularly and successfully linked with the promise of eternal youth, as advertising campaigns emphasized the advantages of being feminine forever – keeping young and retaining unwrinkled skin, firm breasts, and sexual attractiveness generally.

Midway through the 1970s, the popularity of the this treatment fell sharply when it was shown that unopposed estrogen therapy (treatment with estrogen alone) was clearly linked with abnormal cell growth in the endometrium, or lining of the womb, resulting in the likelihood of endometrial cancer. Responding to this evidence, research has concentrated on how to continue the use of estrogen but eliminate the risk of cancer.

As a result of this research, if estrogen alone is administered today, it is given only for three weeks out of four, thus allowing an estrogen-free week. In this fourth week, the stimulation of the endometrium stops, and women may experience bleeding, just like a period, which many find a nuisance. The most favored HRT treatment today is a combination of estrogen and progesterone, one of the progestogen group. Regular bleeding is usually experienced with this regimen.

Progestogens are used because they have the ability to counter-act the adverse effect of estrogen on the endometrium without reducing its favorable effects elsewhere. The protective effect of progestogens is seen to be twofold. First, they promote the shed-ding of the endometrium, which means that the endometrial tis-sue is not allowed to accumulate. Second, progestogens are believed to slow down the actual growth of cells, thus giving further protection against cancer of the womb.

Obviously, clinically speaking, the disadvantages of estrogen therapy described above are relevant only if a woman still has her womb. If the lining of the womb is no longer there, estrogens cannot affect it.

Since estrogen is also known to stimulate breast tissue, cancer of the breast has been another major concern in the administra-tion of HRT. Progestogen supplements are believed to protect the breast from the adverse effect of estrogen buildup. But to date, investigation has been insufficient to assure us absolutely that progestogen used in conjunction with estrogen really does offer a 100 percent guarantee against the risk of cancer.

Who Needs HRT?

The typical HRT recipient has been identified as follows: "The lady who gets treated is a lady who wants to be treated: the lady who has severe symptoms and the lady who has early ovarian failure." (*Siddle*)

If you want to try HRT, then in principle you can seek help from your general practitioner or a gynecologist. If you do not fall into any of the risk categories, then it is likely you will be given the help you require.

Who's at Risk?

We have discussed the most serious side effects of estrogen, but other, less serious side effects can occur. These include nausea, anorexia, vomiting, headaches, and fluid retention leading to weight gain. Estrogens can also aggravate certain illnesses already present; these include high blood pressure, diabetes, migraine, and epilepsy, so estrogen is not recommended for women with a history of these illnesses because of possible adverse drug interactions. Nor is it recommended for women with varicose veins, liver or gall bladder disease, any experience of blood clotting, or cancer in any part of the body, or for women with any history of breast or uterine cancer in the family. Although the link between cancer and estrogen levels has been extensively researched, there is no conclusive evidence about the association between estrogen levels and the effect on the liver, the blood, and the heart, which is why any potential risk of adverse side effects has to be avoided.

A strong candidate for HRT is a woman who, for some reason, experiences ovarian failure in her twenties or thirties. Most gynecologists agree that in this situation a woman should be strongly advised to take estrogen specifically to avoid the accelerated premature bone loss that would otherwise occur within the first five years after the ovaries stop functioning. It is recommended that she take it as soon as possible and for the rest of her life. Long-term estrogen therapy would also be considered for a woman with a strong family history of osteoporosis.

How Do You Take HRT?

HRT is administered by tablets, creams, implants, injection, and adhesive skin patches.

Tablets
The hormone dosage comes in a contraceptive pill–type package, the usual combination being the first two weeks estrogen, the third week estrogen plus progestogen, and the fourth week no tablets at all.

This pill-free week has two consequences. First, the effect of the progestogen will cause a "period," which many women dislike, especially when they feel they have "done away with all that." Second, during this "free" week the estrogen in a woman's bloodstream will fall to its natural level–that is, the level it would normally be without the aid of therapy. This means that she may well experience flushes or sweating in that pill-free week. Again, this is something many women dislike.

For these reasons, standard treatment now often follows a different cyclic pattern involving a combination of pills in which estrogen is administered continuously throughout the twenty-eight days and progestogen is taken for about twelve of those twenty-eight. In this way there is no "free week."

In principle, women should be offered tablets first to be sure they do not react adversely to the type of quantity of the hormones administered. After three months, there is a checkup to deal with any problems. Progestogen-only tablets are also effective in preventing flushes.

Creams

This is the most commonly used form of hormone treatment for a dry vagina, as it can be locally applied. The estrogen acts on the genital membrane to make it thicker and more elastic, increases the cervical secretions within the womb, and makes the vagina less vulnerable to infection and more open to sexual stimulation. Although the estrogen is applied only to the vagina, it is rapidly absorbed through the membrane into the surrounding tissue. "The vaginal estrogen cream is absorbed very well indeed, and it works like a dream." (*McGarry*)

Implants

The same gynecologist explained to us his attitude to HRT implants. "I like to try the two noninvasive methods—pills and creams—first, to find out whether it's going to work. And then I like to move over to the implants. Implants are more convenient for women; they don't have to come back more than three times a year and they don't have problems forgetting to take the pills. Taking pills means 'I'm taking medicine, and therefore I'm ill'; whereas a little implant once every six months is forgotten about within a few days." (*McGarry*)

How does this "little implant" happen?

A tiny pellet of estrogen alone is inserted just under the skin, usually on the lower abdomen or the thigh. Once in place, the pellet stays put, constantly releasing small amounts of hormones automatically as the body needs them, until the total content has been absorbed, probably over a period of three to four months. The whole "operation" needs only a local anesthetic and takes about five minutes.

Unless the woman has had her womb removed she must have the combination of estrogen and progestogen. If the implant is estrogen only, she will be given progestogen supplements to take each month.

So far, the hormones we've discussed have been the female hormones estrogen and progestogen. Another hormone that becomes relevant here is *testosterone*. Essentially, testosterone is the male sex hormone, but some is also produced in women before the menopause.

It is quite common to combine an estrogen implant with one of testosterone, because it is believed to improve the sex drive, and some women find it improves their sense of wellbeing. It is considered beneficial in circumstances where loss of sexual desire is not just a direct result of the discomfort experienced because of a dry vagina.

The generally accepted advantage of implants over tablets is that the hormones go directly into the bloodstream. Like any other substances taken by mouth into the body, estrogens have to be broken down in the liver and the bowel. Some of the substance is passed to the liver, then excreted in the bile to be reabsorbed once more by the intestine. This means, in effect, that some of it passes through the liver twice. So, if there is a history of liver disease, estrogen is not recommended, as it would put unnecessary additional pressure on an already malfunctioning liver. Also, the doses have to be higher when taken by mouth because a lot is lost in the process of digestion and absorption. If it goes directly to the bloodstream without having to go through the stomach first, there is no loss, so the doses can be much lower. This is considered to be one of the main advantages of HRT by implant over other methods.

The primary disadvantage of implants is their inflexibility. Once the implant is in place, you cannot get rid of it until the full six months is up, however badly you react to it. This is why tablets are usually tried at first, to establish the correct dosage of

HRT for each individual woman, so that she is comfortable with it and doesn't suffer any adverse reactions.

Sometimes when a young woman has a total hysterectomy (the ovaries being removed as well as the womb), it is considered appropriate to insert an HRT implant routinely during surgery. This does, however, raise important issues, not the least of which is the lack of informed consent (patient's permission sought and obtained) – hardly possible when the patient is under general anesthesia. The rationale is that it saves time, two jobs being done at once. But there must be real concern, on both ethical and physical grounds, when there is no way of knowing how a particular woman may respond physically or emotionally.

Injection

Estrogen can also be administered in an oily solution by deep intramuscular injection. Although the hormone is rapidly absorbed when given in this way, the rate of absorption afterward can be decreased. It is generally held by the medical establishment to be a less satisfactory method, so HRT by injection is not often recommended.

Patches

The latest method of HRT intake is by means of an estrogen adhesive patch, which is small and made from plastic. One side is semipermeable membrane, which sticks to the skin. Estrogen is contained between this membrane and the patch backing, and is transmitted through the skin into the bloodstream and circulated around the body. There's enough estrogen in the patch to last three days, at the end of which time it has to be replaced. At the time of writing, the patch is still at the experimental stage, but it is expected to be more widely available shortly.

HRT–Assessment and Supervision

Assessment before treatment comprises a comprehensive physical examination, including a Pap smear. If any risk factors are known, then further tests will have to be carried out.

For all women receiving HRT, weight and blood pressure should be checked every six months and a pelvic and breast examination carried out once a year. Cholesterol levels need to be checked every two or three years. Unless you've had a hysterectomy (other than a subtotal hysterectomy), a cervical smear is needed every three to five years, and biopsy of the endometrium annually, whether or not you are experiencing irregular bleeding patterns, or even when you have no vaginal bleeding at all. This may lead to a D and C (scraping) when the lining of the womb is removed under general anesthetic. Alternatively, this can be done in the hospital outpatient department, by use of a suction machine that gently vacuums the inside of the womb. This method causes less pain than a heavy period and is often preferred, as it avoids the necessity for general anesthesia on a fairly regular basis.

Even if you are only using estrogen cream in your vagina, and not taking tablets, the same essential checks should be made. It is a common misunderstanding that because estrogen is applied to the vagina, it somehow stays limited to that area. But estrogen is very easily and rapidly absorbed through the vaginal membrane into the blood and surrounding organs, so a careful watch for abnormal cell growth must be maintained.

How Long Do You Take HRT?

"If you're going to take it, you've got to commit yourself to taking it properly. You can take it for six months, one year, two years, five years, or fifteen years. But you ought to take it properly, rather than messing around missing a tablet here and there, or maybe missing a month at a time, because I don't think it has benefits to do it like that—it's not the way it was designed to work." (*Endacott*)

It is often necessary to use hormone treatment for two to three years. If there are no abnormal symptoms, most doctors will advise you to stop after eighteen months to two years. This is usually done at first by a lower dosage, so that you are slowly weaned off supplementary estrogen.

If you take tablets that follow a pill-free week cycle, you will be encouraged to notice your own reactions during that pill-free week. If, for example, the flushes return in that week, then you may be pleased to start the cycle again. If you find there are no symptoms in that free week, it is a likely indication that your own estrogen levels have reached a point where flushes no longer occur, so you can stop the treatment altogether.

If you are on *continuous* hormone medication, you will be advised to come off it for a couple of months, again to see whether the menopausal symptoms return.

Since no one really knows the scientific cause of hot flushes, it's useful to return to the concept of a "flushing band" (See Chapter 3). This helps to explain why some women stop flushing much sooner than others. It also helps to explain why a woman can be on HRT for ten years and, as soon as she stops, experience hot flushes as distressing as before. If the flushing band theory is correct, it indicates the estrogen has not yet reached a stable level. This is not a common experience, but when it does happen, a woman may well need to remain on estrogen longer, and possibly for the remainder of her life.

Long-term treatment

Other consultants offered reassurance to those women who might have misgivings about long-term treatment. "Well, Mae West was supposed to be taking it when she was eighty-four; I don't know how anecdotal that is, but I see no ill effects for women taking it as long as they want to." (*McGarry*)

"If you have regular blood pressure, you experience regular vaginal bleeding in the pill-free week, your breasts are examined regularly, and you have a regular cervical smear test, there doesn't seem to be any contraindication why a woman should not continue." (*Last*)

Who decides how long?

"Treating a woman at the menopause is a negotiated settlement. It's not a medical prescription in the true sense. How long a woman takes treatment if she comes to me depends on her, not me; there is not reason whatsoever for me to limit treatment." (*Siddle*)

It does seem from our interviews that women themselves make the decision how long to take hormone treatment. "If they push to stay on it, they don't come and ask me to come off it," said Patricia Last. "They just apply for a repeat prescription and they keep hiding. The uptake of HRT in this country is, I think, just 3 percent of the menopausal population; it really is very small."

We interviewed one woman who had been on HRT for twelve years, since the age of forty-nine. She took it because she wanted to avoid menopausal symptoms. She is very happy with it, has regular checkups, and does not anticipate coming off it in the foreseeable future.

Sylvia was offered HRT by her physician for relief of hot flushes. She refused the first time because she didn't like the idea of taking HRT. She saw him again after injuring her shoulder:

"He said to me, 'Now you've done that to your shoulder; for God's sake don't be silly; you really should take this hormone replacement because it will help stop your bones being so brittle.' I did take it and it did take the flushes and sweats away, but I never went back for another batch. I thought, 'Do you go on taking these forever, or what?' I decided to stop and see. I felt very guilty. When he said it would help my bones, I thought that it wasn't about vanity, it was advice. But the idea of taking something chemical to stop the aging process is quite repellent to me."

"From my experience over the years, you'll find that some women will stop coming. They've decided that they want to stop having estrogen treatment and they're going to accept their symptoms. They're doing it of their own volition. I know they're not being told by their physicians to stop, because I work very closely with them." (*McGarry*)

Our own interviews uncovered this kind of self-monitoring, and also some ambivalence towards the medication. "I got the prescription filled," said Doreen, "and then decided that I'd chance it anyway and that I could cope. They went down the toilet eventually." Geraldine said, "I did use estrogen creams and they were absolutely fantastic. But then I got rather worried about them not being safe, so I stopped."

Of our fifteen interviewees, five had received HRT. Of those, four had tablets and one used estrogen cream. Diane took them for three months, and although she felt better, she said, "I don't honestly think it was the pills, I think it was the fact that I brought things out in the open more. My mind told me I was being taken care of."

At the time of interview, Brenda had been taking HRT for her hot flushes, and found it helpful.

Anne suffered hot flushes and sweats and "a terrible draining of confidence." She also suffered from eczema. She found the treatment helped and felt more confident, although she wasn't very happy about the bleeding. At about six months her doctor suggested halving the dose by skipping every other day, intending then to reduce it to one or two tablets a week.

"I tried doing that, and as soon as I started dropping a day I got into an emotional mess. I felt that I couldn't deal with it and went straight back to one a day. Everything cleared up right away. Then after a couple of months I worked away from home for a while and forgot my pills, so I thought, 'Well, this looks like a sign to me, I'll stop them completely this time.' I stopped completely, and everything was fine for nearly a month. And then I was again in a mess, bursting into tears, unable to cope with work, back with hot sweats and some eczema. I phoned my doctor, and this time she sent me a different pill, which makes me bleed more and gives me quite a lot of pain." The whole experience left Anne feeling frustrated: "It's annoying because I don't know what side effects it may have. I'd rather not have to interfere with my system at all, but it damn well helps."

The situation of Sylvia, the member of our group who was persuaded to accept HRT after a shoulder injury, highlights the current increase in offering women HRT to prevent osteoporosis.

HRT Treatment for Osteoporosis

This is where the distinction between specific menopausal symptoms and the effects of normal aging becomes blurred, because short-term treatment cannot be prescribed for osteoporosis as it can for hot flushes. Since our bones become thinner anyway as we age, prevention of this process has to be long-term—ten to fifteen years, starting at the age of fifty.

Experiments show that the acceleration of bone loss after the menopause can be prevented by estrogen therapy. However, although the mechanism involved is not fully understood, once bone loss has occurred, estrogen cannot reverse the process. Estrogen therapy has shown a relative decline in the rate of fractures.

"The reason I don't have a large and highly profitable clinic is because we don't have the means yet available to know who needs to take estrogen. What we need badly is a way that tells us which 25 percent of women are at risk from osteoporosis." (*Siddle*)

The greatest disadvantage of HRT so far discovered is that if estrogens are used for prevention of bone loss and the treatment is interrupted or stopped, no matter how long the treatment has been going on, there follows a disastrous acceleration in loss of bone density. This virtually means that once you have started HRT you have to be on it forever.

In the Western world, the financial consequences of osteoporosis are considerable, and the number of women living after the menopause is always increasing. The estimated cost per year of hip fractures in this group of women is very high; it's hardly surprising, therefore, that estrogen therapy is being promoted as it is, because it can be seen to be an economical measure in terms of preventive health. However, HRT does not constitute a *cure* for osteoporosis–it simply slows the process down.

This issue has been a matter of controversy for the past few years, and alternatives to HRT have been put forward. Calcium, for example, is essential in the maintenance of bone density, and a diet containing plenty of calcium will help maintain bone structure. Vitamins and exercise also help (See Chapter 9).

The HRT Dilemma

There is no doubt in the minds of many doctors and their patients that estrogen has a beneficial effect. Apart from straight relief of symptoms, the overall effect can be astonishing. Speaking of the improvement in a patient, nurse Lysette Butler commented: "It's quite amazing. After treatment, she's gone back to her old self; she's taking care of herself, not so snappy or tired."

"You can see a patient with classic menopausal symptoms, you can give her some treatment and say, 'Come back in a month.'

One month later, a new lady breezes in through the door. She's dyed her hair and has a new outfit and lost weight." (*McGarry*)

Although part of this increased sense of wellbeing must certainly be due to the decrease of symptoms – if you're no longer waking up at night and having hot flashes in the day, and are able to enjoy making love again, it would be difficult not to feel better – it is believed that estrogens have a direct mental tonic effect as well. This has been observed in women who feel wonderful in pregnancy, when the hormone levels change.

A small percentage of women are currently being treated with HRT for menopausal symptoms. From their experience, the general medical opinion is that with assessment and regular supervision, HRT is a good thing, as long as you acknowledge that it isn't a cure-all.

"The fact that your husband is knocking off his secretary can't be treated by prescribing pills. The fact that your aged mother is incontinent and senile and living with you can't be treated by giving you hormones. But the fact you can't sleep at night, that you've got hot flushes, your sexual relationship is deteriorating – those things can be treated and then you're better able to cope with the other problems. You don't stay forever youthful, you don't avoid the other life stresses, you don't avoid mid-life crisis." (*Siddle*)

"Lots of women have social problems at that time – like their children growing up or being troublesome to them, aging parents, husbands insecure at work, financial worries. Estrogen won't help those sorts of problems." (*Butler*)

The arguments or concerns against HRT can be summed up by the phrase *not enough is known*. Although the combination hormone treatment has been shown to reduce the risk of cancer of the endometrium, cancer risks are not completely eliminated. Not enough research has been done to show what the long-term effects of hormone therapy can be, which is of particular concern to those considering taking HRT for the prevention of osteoporosis.

With the emphasis on the withdrawal of estrogen, we can lose sight of the fact that individual levels vary and also that we still have circulating estrogen in our bodies being *naturally* produced. Some estrogen continues to be produced by the ovaries, and some by conversion of a male hormone produced in the adrenal gland. Still more natural estrogen is stored in body fat, from where it is slowly released and metabolized by the liver.

There is also a huge gap in research on men's experience. If more research were carried out on this time in men's lives, it would shed light on which processes are menopausal and which are part of aging. And we cannot ignore the suspicion that now menopause no longer comes within the jurisdiction of psychiatric medicine, it has been taken over by the field of biological medicine. In other words, it is still seen by doctors as a problem. One gynecologist described the menopause as "basic design fault" – in other words, a basic flaw in a woman's body.

From this belief it follows that ideally the fault should be corrected, and in this case, HRT is an obvious way of *bypassing* the fault, thus avoiding all the problems of falling estrogen.

Another common medical view is that the menopause is a crisis and, like any other medical crisis, can be treated with drugs as long as there are no contraindications. And a few other doctors believe that the menopause is "only in the mind," so that HRT will play no part at all in overcoming the problems experienced by some women.

Of course, medical opinion is only a reflection of the culture. The media emphasize the importance of women remaining youthful and attractive to men, and we know that pharmaceutical companies have more to gain by making the menopause into a medical problem needing treatment than by seeing it as a natural transition in any woman's life.

It isn't surprising, with all these pros and cons, that women themselves express a variety of attitudes:

- Some women have no qualms and are very happy to be on HRT for however long is deemed necessary because they feel it suits them.

- Some women are prepared to take HRT as medication for a short while to help them over severe symptoms.

- Some approach HRT with caution, recognizing that they need assistance, but are unhappy about the risks, known and unknown.

- Some women would rather not take medication of any kind, hormonal or otherwise, and prefer to let the menopause run its course naturally.

- Some women suffer distressing symptoms but are unaware that any help is possible, or feel somehow they should endure whatever happens to them at this time in silence.

- Some women experience nothing distressing at all themselves, so the issues surrounding treatment remain completely hypothetical.

In the process of writing this book we discussed the menopause with many women, and several felt their symptoms were serious enough to warrant some attention but were reluctant to be put on HRT. For these women and others who might feel the same, we wrote the next chapter, which deals with homeopathic and herbal treatments. We also look in Chapter 9 at what we can do to help ourselves.

8

Alternatives

———

ORTHODOX medicine works on what is called the allopathic principle. This means that you treat a disease or illness by administering the opposite kind of substance. For example, if your stomach produces too much acid, you take an antacid or alkaline substance to counteract the acidity and to restore a balance.

Homeopathic medicine is based on treating the disease or illness by administering a *similar* substance. A homeopathic practitioner gives a patient naturally prepared medicine that has been tested thoroughly on healthy people to see what symptoms they produce. Instead of treating an illness with an opposite substance, a homeopathic practitioner uses a medicine that if given to a healthy person would elicit the same symptoms. If you have a fever, for example, you would be given a small dose of a substance that if given to a healthy person would produce feverish symptoms. This explains the phrase that describes homeopathic medicines as "treating like with like."

To someone new to homeopathy, this will seem extraordinary. Why, if someone is already suffering, do you give *more* of the same? The answer is that according to homeopathic principles, treating "like with like" stimulates the body's own healing resources to work for themselves. In this way, it is believed that a

patient can be more deeply and completely healed than by allopathic medicine, which can suppress the symptoms and interfere
with the body's natural ability to heal itself.

Consultation

Usually a visit to a physician will last only for minutes. We tend to
be a brief as possible and outline our symptoms objectively, providing a minimum of information, couched in shorthand language
that is more or less medical. For example, you might use the label
"hot flush" rather than describing what it actually feels like as you
experience it. The physician would ask you a few questions about
your periods and your age and, if your answers match certain
criteria, makes a diagnosis, perhaps, that you are menopausal. An
orthodox doctor will look for a cause – in this case, a low level of
estrogen – as an explanation of the symptoms and set out to counteract this situation by raising the level, thus eliminating the
symptom by eliminating the cause.

Consultation with a homeopathic practitioner is lengthy (about
one and a half hours) and very comprehensive. The patient is
asked to give as much information as possible, in detail. At the
first consultation, it may be necessary to ask all sort of questions
relating to family history in order to build up a complete picture of
the person concerned. This is because homeopathy approaches a
patient with a view that includes the person's physical body, of
course, but also the emotions, the mental characteristics, the
temperament, and the general attitude to life. A homeopathic
view of an illness encompasses the whole interaction between all
these different aspects of a human being. A homeopathic practitioner takes all these aspects into consideration when assessing
symptoms. Similarly, you might consider the character of a friend
when trying to understand why that friend behaves in a particular
way. You might look at your friend, and your understanding is
based partly on your friend's personality and partly on the situation to which she is reacting. It is the relationship between *who*
you are and *what* is happening to you that interests the
homeopath.

Symptoms

An orthodox doctor gives treatment for specific symptoms: one thing for influenza, another for diarrhea, something else for a rheumatic knee. This is radically different from homeopathy, which understands the physical symptoms as that particular body's way of responding to an internal change or disturbance. The homeopathic belief is that the physical symptoms are the external signs of the body's internal efforts to defend itself against the disturbance. This is why a homeopathic practitioner doesn't want to suppress the symptoms or control them with drugs, but prefers to stimulate and help the body's defenses to keep up their good work.

Treatment

Homeopathic treatment consists of the application of natural substances obtained from herbal, animal, mineral, and metallic derivatives. They contain no synthetic or unnatural ingredients. These substances work directly on the disturbance in the person in order to correct whatever is out of balance. This allows the body to stop having to cope with the disturbance itself, and so it can cease its efforts. This in turn brings an end to the external symptoms and allows the body to use its energies to heal itself.

Homeopathic preparations are called remedies. Each remedy has a number after it, which indicates the strength or potency of it. The higher the number, the more potent is the remedy, and the more actively it will deal with the disturbance in the person. Each remedy is tested on healthy human volunteers for safety and reliability. The substances are diluted with water or alcohol to control the strength. If you look on the label of a remedy, you will see a figure and then sometimes a letter—an "x," a "D," or a "c"—which indicates the potency.

Most qualified homeopaths believe that lay people should not use potencies above 60x (30c) and that anything more powerful should only be used under the supervision of a homeopathic practitioner.

One of the common beliefs about homeopathic treatment is

that because it is subtle, the medicine is weak and therefore will take ages to work. Our consultant states that in fact, remedies can take effect almost immediately, and that if there has been no effect within twenty-four hours, it is the wrong remedy.

Homeopathy and the Menopause

Homeopathically, menopausal symptoms are seen as a response to fundamental internal changes, an external response that is the best response the woman's body can make in coping with those changes. Treatment for menopausal symptoms therefore addresses itself to the disturbance and helps to redirect the woman's whole being back on course again—rather like returning to the main highway after a detour for road repairs!

If you consult a homeopathic practitioner because you're having hot flushes, you will be asked detailed questions, such as what part of your body is affected, whether the flush is accompanied by sweating, and whether you've noticed any other symptoms that don't appear directly related. For example, you may have found your feet to be incredibly hot at night, or may have noticed an increased desire for salt as well as feeling extra thirsty, or may feel nauseated when you smell food cooking. The homeopathic practitioner divides the symptoms into two categories, general and particular. General symptoms relate to how you feel—for example, "I feel hot," "I feel tearful," "I want to shout," "I have suicidal thoughts," "I feel happy." Particular symptoms are specific experiences such as hot feet or a great thirst. The homeopathic practitioner analyzes all the symptoms together, arranges them in order of importance, and chooses a remedy that fits all the symptoms exactly. If the remedy fits, a cure will take place.

Theoretically this may sound simple—just matching your general and particular symptoms with the clusters of symptoms laid out in the homeopathic manuals. But the accuracy with which a remedy is chosen and its effectiveness depend greatly on the healing skill and insight of the homeopathic practitioner.

If you are interested in this approach or would like to consult a homeopathic practitioner, see the list of organizations at the end of this chapter.

A list of common remedies for menopausal complaints, and some guidelines to help match remedies to symptoms, appears on page 103.

Herbal Medicine

Herbal medicine has been around for many thousands of years and offers another truly natural treatment for severe menopausal symptoms. The substances used are derived from a number of plants, seeds, roots, or barks known for centuries to have had medicinal properties. Many ingredients used in herbal medicines can be found among cooking herbs and spices.

The main advantages of most plant medicines are their low toxicity, lack of accumulation in the body's system, and lack of any side effects. You can't get hooked on herbal medicines, nor do you suffer withdrawal symptoms. Herbal treatment is discontinued once the distressing symptoms disappear and the hormone balance is restored.

We were particularly intrigued to learn from our consultant that she prescribed plants containing substances that encourage the proper production of hormones—a herbal hormone rebalancing therapy. The clover and labiatae families are among these.

An important difference between herbal and orthodox medicine is the extraction of medicinal substances from their original context. For example, dandelion leaves are a potent diuretic, naturally very rich in potassium. Synthetic drug diuretics require potassium supplements. Herbal practitioners prefer to use medicinal plant substances because their natural powerful constituents are perfectly balanced and easily absorbed by the body.

Herbal remedies are very subtle and very potent. As the whole person is taken into consideration when a diagnosis is made, two patients suffering the same symptoms may well be given entirely different substances to suit the differences in personality and symptom experience. So, rather than rushing to buy an over-the-counter remedy that may offer temporary relief, it's much safer and wiser to seek professional guidance from a qualified herbal practitioner, or naturopath, skilled in diagnosing and redressing any permanent underlying imbalance or serious disease.

The herbalist examines and evaluates the patient as a whole person; the emphasis is on realigning the overall temporary imbalance of both mind and body. Like the homeopathic practitioner, he or she will take a long and detailed physiological and psychological case history before prescribing an individual course of treatment.

Herbal remedies can be prescribed in several different ways. The most usual are a liquid tincture, pills, powders, infusions of dried herbs, or local ointments or liniments. Following the initial consultation, your progress will be carefully monitored and supervised every two weeks and the necessary adjustments made to the prescription.

In our consultant herbalist's experience, very often just correcting a patient's diet significantly improves and alleviates many of the distressing symptoms. Junk foods high in nitrates (e.g., salami, ham), wheat, and carbohydrate are common culprits. Too much meat, and—even more remarkably in these days of nutritional awareness—overenthusiastic and uninformed vegetarianism resulting in too little protein, may also cause menopausal difficulties. More exercise and a change from a stressful lifestyle are common recommendations. A frequent contributor to severe menopausal symptoms is the contraceptive pill, because it overrides the natural function of the pituitary gland. Once the pituitary gland has been upset in this way, it's often more difficult to reset the hormonal imbalance. In our herbal practitioner's experience, women who have been on the pill, whether for two months or ten years, can experience more severe hot flushes and flooding than those who opted for alternative methods of contraception.

On average, herbal treatment for the most common and severe menopausal symptoms usually takes about three to six months to rebalance.

The following organizations publish directories of licensed health professionals in their respective fields. Please write or call for information.

The American Association of Naturopathic Physicians
P.O. Box 33046
Portland, OR 97233
503/255-4860

The American Holistic Medical Association/Foundation
2727 Fairview Avenue East
Seattle, WA 98102
206/322-6842

The International Foundation for Homeopathy
2366 Eastlake Avenue East, Suite 301
Seattle, WA 98102
206/324-8230

The National Center for Homeopathy
1500 Massachusetts Avenue, N.W.
Suite 41
Washington, DC 20005
202/223-6182

9

Help Yourself

———

MOST of the help we've described so far has come from other people, professionals of orthodox and alternative medicine, and concerned individuals outside the medical profession. In this chapter we take a look at the equally important part you can play in looking after yourself and in encouraging other women to help themselves.

"Like any other aspect of health care, a woman's experience of her symptoms during and after the menopause can be helped by taking better care of herself" (*Siddle*)

"If you can adopt a positive attitude to health at this age you're going to have a much happier life." (*McGarry*)

"If you ask me if there are ways in which you can minimize the effects of ovarian failure without recourse to medication, the answer is 'Yes.' But you can't increase your estrogen production by thought alone. At least if you can, I'm not aware of it." (*Siddle*)

Our individual level of estrogen production varies enormously, as we have explained, but we can help ourselves by avoiding smoking and excess alcohol, because these cause the estrogen in our bodies to be broken down and used up at a faster rate. Cutting down on coffee or tea and hot spicy foods can help to

76

prevent making hot flushes worse, as will wearing looser clothing, especially around the neck.

It's also important to be able to relax, a point stressed by Rosie.

"Every time we meet we have half an hour's relaxation first. I find that all the women who come through my group say how helpful it's been. Now, when they go to bed, when they're tossing and turning, they just either put the tape on or go through the relaxation themselves."

Most women interviewed were conscious of their diet and tried to follow a healthy regimen, allowing for occasional indulgences.

We do not have the space to give you more than a basic introduction to a healthy diet, but you can learn more about the benefit of nutrition and vitamins by reading several of the many books now available on the subject.

Diet

Diet is extremely important during and after the menopause. Women after menopause tend to suffer the same rate of cardiovascular disease as men of the same age, because of losing the protective effect of estrogen. A good diet contributes effectively to a reduction in heart and blood vessel problems and, according to some experts, can help to prevent or contain the development of cancer.

A sensible well-balanced diet containing esential vitamins and minerals can help us adapt and adjust more easily to the changes going on in our bodies in the years leading up to and after the menopause. Keep your meals as simple as possible. Eat more uncooked fruits, salad vegetables, lightly steamed vegetables, skim milk, butter, wheat germ, nuts and raisins, cheese, eggs, and lightly grilled fish.

Cut out white flour products, sugar, dried foods, cooked cereals, puffed or toasted breakfast cereals, tea, coffee, jam, pastry, cookies, candy, processed meats such as sausage and salami, and fried potatoes.

We can function normally and happily if we ensure that we have enough calcium; vitamins D, E, B-complex, and C; magnesium; iron; and iodine in our daily diet, so there's no need to overdose on megavitamins!

Protein

Protein is important for healthy skin, nails, hair, muscles, brain, internal organs, and bones.

Highest sources of protein: Skim milk, wheat germ, unprocessed cheeses, and eggs.

Calcium

The best weapon in the fight against osteoporosis and brittle bones is physical exercise and an adequate calcium intake, Our daily recommended intake of calcium at menopause is 1000–1500 mg.

Our calcium level must be delicately balanced against proper amounts of vitamin D to ensure that the calcium is absorbed by the intestine; we also need magnesium, which ensures that the calcium stays in the bones and is not excreted. However, some calcium-rich foods are high in phosphorus, and too much phosphorus actually draws calcium from the bones, so we should avoid eating excessive amounts of phosphorus-rich products such as turkey, ham, pork, fried potatoes, bread, processed meats, crackers, and soft drinks.

As a rough guide, our daily calcium intake should be twice that of magnesium and equal to that of phosphorus.

Foods rich in calcium: Skim milk; cottage, cream, and hard cheeses; low-fat yogurt; canned salmon and sardines (calcium in the edible bones); raw oysters; shrimp; cooked scallops; dark green leafy vegetables such as broccoli, lettuce, raw watercress, and cabbage; celery; peanuts; walnuts; sunflower seeds; dried beans; tahini (creamed sesame seed, which is higher in calcium than skim milk); wheat germ; soy flour; dates; cauliflower; dried fruit; chicory; fennel; leeks; parsley; raw parsnips; sweet potatoes.

Highest natural sources of vitamin D: Butter, egg yolk, liver, soft or hard margarine, D–enriched skim milk, shrimp, mackerel, sardines, herring, salmon, tuna. Sunlight is another natural source of vitamin D.

Foods rich in magnesium: Bran, brazil nuts, wheat germ, almonds, soy flour, peanuts, millet, whole wheat flour, walnuts, oatmeal.

Essential Vitamins

Vitamin E

Improves the skin and blood flow, prevents clotting and vaginal irritation. *But handle it with care.* Especially if you have high blood pressure, diabetes, or a rheumatic heart condition, never take vitamin E supplements unless supervised by a physician.

Highest natural sources: Cottonseed, corn, soybean, safflower, wheat germ, coconut, peanut, and olive oils. Wheat germ, apple seeds, alfalfa, barley, dried soybeans, peanuts, rosehips, yeast, cabbage, spinach, asparagus, whole wheat bread.

Vitamin C + Rutin (Bioflavin)

Helps avoid rheumatism, arthritis, and the buildup of bacteria in the joints and kidneys (200–500 mg daily).

Highest natural sources: Oranges, broccoli, brussels sprouts, strawberries, cabbage, red peppers.

Vitamin B and B_6

Helps alleviate nervous disorders (5–10 mg daily).

Highest natural sources: Wheat germ, brown rice, bran, soy flour, brewers' yeast, ham, asparagus, watercress, liver, kidneys, brain, heart, spinach, chicken, kale, sweet potatoes, corn on the cob, whole-grain cereals, molasses, walnuts, peanuts, herring, salmon, bananas, avocados, grapes, pears, cabbage, carrots, egg yolks, sardines, crab, oysters, cheese (soft, hard, and cream).

Other Minerals

Iodine

Good for the thyroid gland; improves general vitality and hair and scalp condition; prevents constipation, weight gain, and depression.

Highest natural sources: Dark green vegetables, lettuce, spinach, grated carrot, beets, parsley, and celery. (See also kelp, in mineral supplements below.)

Iron

Vital ingredient of the red pigment in the blood. Iron deficiency is signaled by lack of appetite, dizzy spells, headaches, and poor memory. Non–meat eaters will need vitamin C for efficient absorption of iron (24 mg daily).

Highest source of organic iron: Liver, wheat germ, whole wheat flour, oatmeal, brown rice, parsley, prunes, carrots, raw celery, raw onions, apples, bananas, cherries, dates, grapes, orange and lemon juices, peaches, pears, pumpkins, mushrooms, raisins, honey, molasses, canned salmon, sardines, raw cabbage, lettuce, soybeans, cooked potatoes, spinach, pineapple, and tomatoes.

Mineral Supplements in Tablet Form

Kelp
Powdered kelp contains iodine plus iron, copper, calcium, phosphorus, potassium, sulfur, sodium, magnesium, manganese, chlorine, cobalt, boron, and barium—adding up to the best source of the multiminerals and trace elements we need in our daily diet.

Magnesium with calcium
Prevents restlessness, muscle tremor, irritability, and overexcitability; helps calcium stay in the bones.

Ginseng

Useful tonic, energizer, and "mystical medicine"–its botanical family name *Panax* means "panacea," or cure-all. Although the mechanism is still not yet fully understood, the ginseng root contains substances that can control hormone levels in the body. Ginseng with vitamin E has been used to alleviate hot flushes, night sweats, nervous tension, headaches, palpitations, mild depression, insomnia, and lack of sexual desire. But make sure you get the whole root extract, undiluted and not mixed with anything else. Buy it only from a reputable health store or pharmacy (400–600 mg dried root daily).

Royal Jelly

Royal jelly allegedly contains a substance that stimulates estrogen production; it also contains vitamin B complex and is often mixed with bee pollen (300 mg dried royal jelly daily). We don't know exactly how effective it is in relieving menopausal symptoms, nor do we know about the possible risk involved in taking it, but Barbara Cartland is rumored to have been taking royal jelly for years!

Finally, at the end of a busy day, why not try a herbal tea?

Camomile Flowers and Valerian Root

These are popular herbal sedatives.

Evening Primrose Oil

At the dosage of one or two 500-mg capsules taken three times daily, this oil can help control menopause symptoms because of its role in prostaglandin synthesis. These, in turn, can help the flagging estrogen production by the body.

Exercise

"There are quite a few women in their fifties who never do anything. I see them just sitting around. For menopausal women, exercise is terribly important. It strengthens the bones if you take vigorous exercise at least once a week and also stimulates the adrenal gland." (*McGarry*)

"I actually exercise more than I have done in the past. I stretch more, dance or something. I like to keep loose but I don't do enough." (*Bea*)

"I like exercise such as swimming but I despise running. It must have something to do with having short legs!" (*Lisa*)

"I manage to walk every day and I've got a bicycle now." (*Brenda*)

Even if you can discipline yourself to just twenty minutes of exercise three times per week, your body will benefit. It need not be a chore, so choose an activity you enjoy.

Special Exercises for a Special Muscle

However eagerly you jog, swim, or dance, there is one muscle that you won't exercise in these ways. This is the "pc" muscle. This stands for *pubococcygeal*, because the muscle stretches from your pubic bone in front to your coccyx, or tailbone, behind. Some women are introduced to this muscle as the pelvic floor muscle when preparing for childbirth. Many women in Asian cultures are introduced to the importance of this muscle as a routine part of growing up to be a sexual adult, but in the West this is overlooked.

This is the muscle that contracts in orgasm, so exercising it can certainly help your sexual response and enjoyment. The reason for including it here, however, is that the following exercises increase the blood flow to your genitals; this helps to keep the vagina moist and healthy.

The exercises are known as Kegel exercises, so called for the doctor who designed them for his middle-aged women patients who were suffering from incontinence. These women apparently reported not only relief from the original problem but increased enjoyment of sexual activity as well. You could try the following:

- First identify the muscle: imagine yourself in the midst of urinating and then having to stop suddenly. The muscle you clench to stop is the pc muscle.
- Once you've found it, slowly contract it in as far as you can and then let it go. Do this to a count of three seconds. Contract, draw it in – 1, 2, 3 – and let it out – 1, 2, 3. Repeat this a few times.

- Next, try fluttering the muscle. This means not contracting it fully, all at once, but just taking it in a little way and letting it go quite quickly. The effect feels like a fluttering around the vagina.

- Finally, do the more advanced exercise, called "the elevator" because you imagine you are contracting the muscle in six stages as the lift climbs up six floors. When you reach "the top floor," hold the contraction for a couple of seconds before letting it out again slowly down each floor to the ground. Contract slowly: first floor, second floor, and so on up to the sixth—hold it—and then slowly let the muscle go with each count downward.

These exercises are easy to do, and they can be done sitting, standing, or lying down—anytime, any place. You can use the time during a boring meeting or waiting in line at the supermarket quite constructively, and no one will be any the wiser!

Skin Care

Several of our interviewees reported taking special care of their skin to counteract the dryness. Caroline said she never used soap in the bath but preferred "one of those nice foam conditioning oils," Bea had started using glycerine soap, and Mary opted for honey lotion on her face and arms. Brenda had gone on using cocoa butter on her feet and hands every night, as she had always done. Diana described another personal ritual.

'I do something for myself every day. I've always massaged my body after my shower. Something for every area; it's a habit. It's an inheritance from my mother: she used to do it with oatmeal and lemon."

Maybe forming such a habit makes it easier to look after our bodies, because several women reported that although the spirit is willing, the flesh is often too weak. "What I think and what I do are two different things," one of them said. "I think exercise is absolutely vital, but I don't do much!" Another, echoing this, said "I know what I should be doing and I probably will, but I'm not doing it right *now*; that's my problem!"

"Everyone tells me, 'More exercise,' but it's work, you know. At a time when you want to relax and put you feet up but you can't, you've got to keep yourself well-oiled." (*Angela*)

It's important to care for our bodies inside and out. But we have to persuade ourselves that we're important enough. Advice and suggestions will have no impact if we do not basically believe that we're worth it. A lifetime's habit can be easy enough to maintain, but during the menopause, as at other times of change in our lives, we need to give ourselves *extra* care.

A woman's relationship with her body can change at this time; she may feel herself less attractive. She may simply find it disconcerting that her shape is changing. "The thing that most profoundly affected me is my change in body shape," said Jo. "I still find it difficult to come to terms with."

Sometimes we need reassurance.

"My belly has become really podgy, and I can remember being self-conscious when I was naked with J. I said so and he was very loving." (*Bea*)

Our bodies lose their familiarity. No longer having a recognizable cycle, from month to month, with predictable ups and downs, we can lose our sense of rhythm and for this reason can feel less confident and stable.

"You don't know what your body's going to do from day to day. And because you've always been identified with your body, you know that it matters. It's you. And you have to ask yourself what your relationship with your body has been and what it's going to be. You do feel very vulnerable." (*Angela*)

We need to keep in touch with our bodies.

"I always say to my classes, 'You've got to tell your brain that your ovaries are stopping functioning; so your brain has to relearn as well. We've all got to work together and learn about what's happening. We've got to listen to our bodies because your body can educate you and you can educate your body.'" (*Rosie*)

Taking the time to look after your body properly is crucial, even if you feel you're being self-indulgent. "I really had to start loving my body all over again," Angela said; "I suppose because of the feeling other people might not. But it felt essential."

Talking It Through

So far we've looked in detail at how we can take care of our bodies *inside*. We also need to explore ways in which we can take better care of ourselves on the *outside*—in other words, consider how to communicate what we feel and what we fear, in a way that will bring us both emotional and practical support when we need it.

One of the best ways to cope with any stress is to talk about it. A couple of our interviewees did not feel the need to talk to anyone, because their menopause was experienced without difficulty. The remainder of the group indicated that whereas in other situations a woman might have found it relatively easy to discuss problems and anxieties with a friend, on the subject of menopause silence often reigned.

"I really didn't discuss it because I wasn't concerned about it. I just mentioned it to close people like my mother and sister." (*Doreen*)

"One of the things I find most unhelpful is that most of my friends have completely denied they have had any problems at all. It's only when I've really challenged them I found they *did* have symptoms but completely sat on them." (*Anne*)

Why do we keep so quiet? Is it fear of being unfairly stereotyped?

"I never spoke about it, I thought they'd think it slightly ridiculous, and that if one made a big deal of menopause, then you'd suddenly be thought of as someone whose whole life was bound up in their biology." (*Sylvia*)

"It's all to do with being nothing but a sex object. If the menopause finishes you as a sex object, then it finishes you as a person and you can't admit it's happening. So having got through it without difficulty is seen as some sort of badge, which declares I've managed it all with grace and dignity and without losing any of my sex appeal." (*Anne*)

Brenda found it easy to talk with other women of the same age: "With friends of my own age we've all talked about it. I seem to be the only one in my circle that seems to have had hot flushes, funnily enough."

At the time of the interview, Bea described herself as premenopausal. But she had already initiated conversations at work and very much appreciated the value of sharing with other women. "Particularly at work but in some of our regular get-togethers, it's been really good hearing other women talk about their experiences, actually to have the truth, to get rid of some of the myths and horror stories."

Several years after Diana's menopause, she found that younger women wanted to talk to her. "I know now what a lot of people experience, particularly the depression, and I know it's just a development. It's because you are on your own and because no one understands. Many of them express lack of confidence, saying, 'I'm not myself,' and I say, 'Yes, I felt like that; yes, I did exactly that'; there are exactly the same behavior patterns again and again."

Anne, too, is convinced of the value of talking honestly with other women. "Many women think it's an achievement to have been through without any problems. I've gone through kicking and screaming, so I think what is most helpful is to come up against somebody who is also finding it difficult and is not afraid to say so."

Apart from talking with other women for reassurance, which can itself alleviate much of the stress, there is a further dimension to encouraging communication at this time—and that's talking to those we live with, especially if we want them to help.

"If you don't convey how you feel to the family that's living with you, if you don't tell them, then they're not going to know, so how can they help?" (*Rosie*)

Give Yourself a Break

One of the biggest stumbling blocks to asking for practical help appears to be a feeling of guilt. Unfortunately, it is often said that the husband or family of a menopausal women bears the brunt of her erratic behavior. This means she either voluntarily goes to the doctor because she's feeling guilty, or is sent there with instructions to sort herself out. It's difficult to imagine a more unfair situation than a woman being criticized because she can't cope with the amount of stress in her life. "It's much more important to accept that they are reacting in a completely *normal* way. It's understandable, not irrational." (*Last*)

And yet, far worse than any criticism from outside is the way in which we constantly blame ourselves for failing to keep up with the superwoman image. This image exhorts us to be ever-giving, ever-coping, and ever-strong, and when we fall short we feel terribly inadequate. It's just this feeling of failure that makes us shy away from asking for the help from others that would make life so much easier.

"I learned going to the group that I should give in to those feelings a little more, find space for myself, and forget the housework. Because there'll come a day when I'll feel like doing it and get through it. If I didn't feel like cooking a meal at the weekend, I'd tell the family, 'I don't feel like cooking; if you want something, you do it.' And I did it, and it worked and I felt much more able to cope." (*Rosie*)

It can be easy for us at any age to become so absorbed with other people's needs that we neglect our own. But with what is likely to be happening in the lives of middle-aged women, this tendency to become a magnet for other people's concerns can be quite self-destructive. "Women in their early fifties are like Atlas; they carry the world on their shoulders. Some of the women who come to see me have so many of other people's burdens, they barely have time to concern themselves with their own." (*Siddle*)

When we asked this gynecologist what he would advise in this circumstance, he replied, "Stop being such good listeners—tell the world to bug off!" If you think that's a bit drastic, remember the importance of getting some balance between your needs and those of other people. The key to this is valuing yourself enough to see that whoever else is making demands in your life, you have a right to have some time for yourself.

"After the course, women go away with the start of self-esteem; they do all sorts of things in the household, making small changes to claim some time and space for themselves." (*Jo*)

"I pass this information on to my ladies. They must try and give themselves half an hour off every day and also arrange half a day during the week that they can have to themselves. They can do what they want to do—stay in bed for that half a day, or go out for a walk and look around the stores. Anything that suits them. It certainly helps. You've *got* to educate your family or those around you to this different way of life." (*Rosie*)

Instead of repeatedly criticizing ourselves, we could perhaps try a little self-praise, especially if we have to put a lot of effort into looking after others at the same time as going through our menopause. "Many women have elderly relatives or other dependents they're looking after at home—it's a great strain and nobody tells them they're doing a marvelous job." (*Last*)

For women in this situation, this gynecologist prescribed plenty of tender loving care. Certainly, getting this from others is important, but never underestimate the value of giving it to yourself. Loving yourself is:

- Putting your feet up and asking for a cup of tea.
- Looking in the mirror with pride.
- Crying when you want to.
- Enjoying closeness with another person.
- Reading about your body.
- Watching what you put inside your body.
- Stretching it fully.
- Saying it hurts when it does.
- Letting yourself be ratty without giving yourself a hard time.

- Having a long luxurious soak in the bath with special bath oil.
- Saying "Yes, it's my menopause" with a big smile.
- Exercising for pleasure.
- Singing, breathing deeply, laughing.
- Saying "No" when you want to.
- Telling a friend how you really feel.
- Resting—*before* you are on your knees!

10

Men and the Menopause

COPING with male attitudes, whether in society at large, in the home, workplace, or all three, can create extra stress for a woman during her menopause. "When one talks to men about the menopause, one gets almost complete blankness, because there is often so little awareness of what it is. It isn't actually something that's on their level of consciousness." (*Siddle*)

"They're uneasy with it because they don't completely understand it. So therefore it's alien. They don't want to face the situation, because it's feelings and emotions, and men don't particularly like feelings. They don't want to get into that level of it." (*Diana*)

We are often aware of existing stereotypes:

"I think that men feel, when women are entering their late forties and fifties, that they're irrational, and they put that down to the fact they're going through that time of life." (*Doreen*)

"Irrational" is a familiar label attached to women by those men who find emotional behavior difficult to understand at the best of times; at the menopause this stereotype reaches its height.

"Everybody's frightened of being considered a menopausal nut, you know." (*Last*)

It's true that our behavior and feelings can be difficult to explain even to ourselves, let alone to anyone else. And even if you do begin to understand what's happening in your body, will others be able to? Sometimes men find the whole subject of "women's things" very uncomfortable to think or talk about. Doreen felt this was truer of men in their sixties and over, but felt that younger men were more tolerant.

If a man is embarrassed he will be unlikely to ask for information. "An extremely common complaint a woman will make is 'My husband is very good, very understanding, but he doesn't understand this sort of thing.'" (*Siddle*)

When Diana talked to her husband, he said "You'd better see the doctor." But Maureen and Brenda described their husbands as easygoing and understanding about the whole thing, especially in being able to make light of the subject yet be supportive when their wives had hot flushes.

But Brenda was puzzled by her reaction when, although her relationship with her teenage son was very open, she still felt unable to tell him exactly what was going on. "He said to me the other week, 'Mother, you're bathed in perspiration; I've never noticed you so hot before.' So I said to my husband, 'Go and tell him, he's *your* son.'" Angela didn't talk to her teenage sons either. She felt they would neither understand nor be interested, and didn't want to burden them.

Maybe one of the reasons why we don't speak up is related to Bea's insight. "I've never had a direct conversation with my husband about it. I might say something about getting older or link that in with having my period or a severe headache. But it's always oblique, never direct. I think it's because there's a bit of me that really doesn't want to say to him, 'Well, you know, I'm getting older.' There's that bit of me that still wants to be younger."

It can be difficult to avoid the negative bias of stereotyped thinking, especially from colleagues at work.

"I believe men would not employ women at that age if they had a choice. They would tend to shy away from it because they think it would create problems." (*Doreen*)

It can put extra strain on a woman who feels she must therefore avoid these assumptions. "I would put on a brave face at work," recalled Rosie. "I had to meet reps and go out on the shop floor because I was the assistant buyer."

"You're sitting quietly in court with two men and you're all hot and bothered, and they turn to you and you feel terrible because everyone's looking at you." (*Brenda*)

And even working with other gynecologists doesn't appear to grant a woman immunity.

"They say to me, if I get very cross about something, 'Oh come on Pat, settle down, you're having a hot flush you know.' I get so cross about it. You bend over backwards to try to be this kind of stereotyped lady. And it's so difficult." (*Last*)

You can still be vulnerable to negative associations even if you are a medical expert. Although Sheila was actually teaching the menopause to her nursing students, she found it "too close to home" to be able to refer to her own experience as an example. "I suppose I'm still hanging on to the idea nobody knows I'm menopausal and they still think I'm normal and that I haven't yet reached that age."

Obviously, one can't guarantee that information will wipe away prejudice, but Doreen, as a personnel manager, was very eager to have information made more available at work.

"I would like a simple leaflet that one could hand out to managers, most of whom are men. It should contain the sorts of things that can happen and the possible reactions, and say there is a way of dealing with them. For example, if you are in a meeting and you could see that one of your female colleagues is in a little distress, rather than making either a major production or just ignoring it, you could maybe suggest that you "have a natural break," that "this is a good time to stop," or "let's get a cup of coffee," so that the person can withdraw discreetly, tidy herself up, make herself feel more comfortable, and come back into the meeting. It's more important that they (men) become sensitized to the outward signs of a distressed colleague, so that if you see someone get emotional, you know how to handle it. You know not to create more stress and anxiety for that person but instead be supportive. This type of information I feel would be a great asset for managers and colleagues, because there are days when you're close to tears and even the silliest thing can start you weeping. People need to be aware of that."

A Man's Own Changes

If a man is himself experiencing changes at middle age, this is likely to affect his attitude to a woman in a similar position.

"I don't think they're actively thinking, 'You're finished.' But it brings them back to themselves again. They're the same age, so if it's happening to you they may not want to know that it's happening to them as well. It's just that they don't have anything visible. I think men ignore it whereas women face up to it, and I think women are put down more because of it." (*Diane*)

"Men can behave totally irrationally and no one says, 'He's just having a hot flush today.' It's very easy for men to put down their own fears. If his wife has an affair he won't say, 'I can't satisfy my wife sexually'; he'll say, 'She's gone a bit nympho in the menopause.' He'll always try and turn it around.' (*Last*)

So is the male menopause a myth itself or reality? One of our consultants said flatly, "Men don't menstruate, so male menopause is a nonsense." (*Siddle*)

"A lot of men would not accept the idea that they go balmy, and they insist they're very sane. But dealing with so many men at work, I'm sure I can spot signs of male menopause." (*Senanayake*)

"When you're talking about a man who's going through problems they talk about the 'midlife crisis.' For women it's 'that time of her life.'" (*Doreen*)

Obviously, men can't stop menstruating, but they can experience hormonal changes. This is more correctly known as the male climacteric and has been defined as a combination of physical, psychological, and hormonal changes that are accompanied by a reduction in sexual activity.

Overall, the male climacteric has a much lower profile than the female climacteric, partly because the changes are not as marked, nor can they be linked to such an obvious and specific cut-off point as a woman's last period. Yet, there is a general acceptance that men after the age of fifty-five, and often earlier, experience a variety of symptoms that affect their attitudes to society and to their own lifestyle. These include irritability; difficulty in concentrating; decreased sexual desire; some depression; and withdrawn, antisocial behavior.

In 1980, a survey among male and female patients in an Oxford physician's practice indicated several parallel experiences. Both men and women were asked to respond to questions related to middle age. Research has also shown that physical changes can be a part of the male climacteric. Bone loss starts at about sixty (ten years later than in women), and density declines steadily but at a slower rate. Skin changes such as loss of elasticity are noticed in men, and in a few men, an experience similar to hot flushes can occur.

Although there is a widely held belief that the male climacteric is due solely to cultural and psychological factors, it is certain that men experience hormonal decline. Testosterone, produced in the testicles, begins to fall in many men after the mid-forties and in the vast majority after sixty. Testosterone is described as the hormone of sexual libido in both men and women, which is why, as we described in Chapter 7, it can be administered in implant form to women who seek medical help for lack of sexual desire.

Research also shows that sexual activity declines with age. This is measured in loss of potency; that is, a man finds it difficult to get a full erection so that he can enter his partner's vagina, or he finds he can get an erection but loses it easily. This of course happens to most men at some time in their lives, but as they get older it becomes much more pronounced.

It is difficult for a man to avoid the cultural conditioning that measures maleness in terms of virility—that you are only a man if you can achieve penetration. Therefore it is not surprising that loss of sexual potency can be accompanied by lack of self-confidence, fatigue, and depression. A few men seek medical help for this problem and are given extra male hormones to boost their own lowered level. But fear of cancer of the prostate (a small gland behind the bladder) has prevented widespread use of testosterone for men.

Most of our interviewees were aware of a cultural double standard in attitudes to age. A man's attractiveness can be enhanced with age, whereas women feel their attractiveness wanes. Yet, the phenomenon of the middle-aged man discarding his wife of thirty years for a younger, and therefore considered more attractive, woman is not unusual, and this must indicate an underlying sexual insecurity.

A further insecurity is related to the second major aspect of man's conditioning: his achievement in the workplace. In a society like ours today, where loss of one's job is an ever-present threat, middle age can also bring a further psychological blow to a man's sense of identity.

This consideration of men's experience of their middle age raises some interesting questions that reflect on cultural attitudes to a woman's experience.

Apart from the information about sexual performance, very little is known about changes in men at this time of life. Given that physical changes occur in men, too, why is there not more research to determine how widespread this experience is? We would then be a lot clearer about the changes related to the human aging process as distinct from those related specifically to the menopause. And why it is apparently so easy to accept male changes as a combination of psychological, social, and hormonal changes, while female changes are seen as almost exclusively a result of *hormonal* change?

This leads us to ask a further question: Why does the risk of prostate cancer prevent widespread administration of testosterone to men, while estrogen is widely recommended for administration to women, even though the cancer risks have not been completely eliminated? Is it considered easier to more profitable to experiment widely on women? If so, the implications are profound.

It's interesting to speculate about why the menopause has become a medical problem in women but not in men. If men are moody, irrational, irritable, or antisocial, do they feel ashamed enough to seek medical help from a doctor to restore their good humor? In the absence of informed answers to all these questions, we can only invite you to draw your own individual conclusions!

11

Onward and Upward

"THIS whole thing of what is menopausal and what is midlife or aging is a bit of an open question." (*Last*)

"Depending how you're aging anyway, the menopause will coincide with your continuing aging process. Men don't suddenly age and women don't suddenly age because of the menopause. Menopause is just really a convenient hook to hang the aging process from." (*Jo*)

"If you take a woman who takes estrogen, that doesn't stop her getting wrinkles; it doesn't stop her getting old. Whether or not she adjusts to the aging process is a different issue." (*Siddle*)

In this part of the world, a woman after the normal age of menopause (around fifty-one) has an average life expectancy of a further twenty-five years—in other words, the next third of her life. Strictly speaking, we're aging every minute after birth, but from our forties onward, and sometimes earlier, we begin to recognize signs of getting older: slowing down; maybe feeling more self-confident; not being able to take late nights; feeling more tolerant, less radical, or maybe less fit than we used to. The occasional gray hair, loosening skin, changing eyesight—all these little signs are part of a gradual changing process, which accelerates in later years.

Although the menopause isn't exactly a trigger to aging, it does act as a convenient marker in women's lives. Certainly, as has already been described, one of the fears about acknowledging the fact of being menopausal is the implication that a corner has been turned – that you are somehow "over the hill." But physiologically this isn't true.

There isn't a sudden change, but turning fifty does seem to be a milestone. Since we live in a society that is self-conscious about age, and where the premium is on qualities of sleekness, speed, and dispensability, it's not surprising that aging is a constant undercurrent in any discussion about menopause. That is why we decided to include it in this book.

Aging is often what other people see you doing; it's not necessarily what you see in yourself.

"I was told in a clothes shop that those clothes were a bit young for me. It was an absolute shock; I though they can't be talking about me!" (*Geraldine*)

"I'm not afraid of being old, because I don't feel old inside. It's just a nasty shock when you see an old lady in the mirror opposite and find it's you. (*Mary*)

"You just think you'll go on the same as you are, it's only when you catch sight of yourself that you realize." (*Diana*)

And what exactly is *old* anyway?

"I used to think 'sixty' but not that I'm sixty, I know I'm not there yet. It's always ahead of you. *Other* people are old." (*Diana*)

"Old is five years older than I am and it keeps growing." (*Sylvia*)

"Probably sixty-five. A point at which crucial parts of one's consciousness start to fail, needing help from other people." (*Lisa*)

"When I was younger I though fifty was old; now I think that seventy is old. What would be old for me would be if I gave up paid work; then I really would move into that time." (*Geraldine*)

"I think over fifty is the crucial thing. Maybe because it's your chance to start and take control of what you are going to do, because if you haven't sorted it out by the time you're sixty, you're just going to let it go." (*Angela*)

"There's this sadness that you're suddenly confronted with the fact you are getting older. The older you get the further away it gets. I suppose I'd say 'over seventy' was old." (*Sheila*)

What do you notice physically?

"The extent to which you misuse your body is the most fundamental criterion of the extent and rate at which you will age." (*Jo*)

"I'm a bit physically slower, I don't do things as quickly. I could do a room in an hour; now I make it take all day; I don't rush any more." (*Diana*)

"One of the problems I've had has been trouble with my joints and legs. That's the kind of place where you get old in your body. You shouldn't, you mustn't, and yet you do." (*Angela*)

"My pubic hair getting white; that's something I don't like very much." (*Geraldine*)

Several women also mentioned that their eyesight was changing.

Anticipation

How do we anticipate getting older?

"I hope that as I get older, I can let go of possessions. I shall enjoy my grandchildren; I don't have to feel I'm responsible for them but can love and respect them." (*Geraldine*)

"I'll have to leave behind being flirtatious and be a sensible, wise old woman. But I don't know how to do it." (*Lisa*)

"I've always had a philosophy that today is the most important day, and I want to enjoy it. I can't do anything about getting older, so there's no point in worrying about it." (*Doreen*)

"I'm afraid of getting nearer to death, but I've never minded the years passing. You know, that sort of tick, tick, tick, as my age goes up! I haven't minded that." (*Anne*)

"I have a horror of looking at some of the older single women who live around here. They look like chronic invalids. Gray—so gray." (*Angela*)

"An awareness of your own mortality." (*Diana*)

"My mother suffers from senile dementia, and that worries me terribly. So if ever I forget anything and the family say, 'You're just like your mother,' it's like a red rag to a bull because it really goes home. They say it in fun but it's horrendous. I couldn't bear to be like that." (*Sheila*)

Although we know that aging is natural and inevitable, we are encouraged to delay it as long as possible, especially as women.

"If you're a sixty-five-year-old woman, and you want to think, act, and look like a fifty-five-year-old, you need to take estrogens. You might well be a sixty-five-year-old woman who is well able to keep her act together. But the majority of untreated sixty-five-year-olds will obviously be different from their fifty-five-year-old counterparts. They will have loss of muscle tone, loss of bone, loss of collagen (the protein that keeps your skin glowing and youthful) visible to any observer. They are much less likely to be sexually active, even if they want to be." (*Siddle*)

This medical practitioner's statement reflects exactly what women face in this culture: the unfavorable comparison with younger women and the exclusive emphasis on our appearance as a measure of our sexual viability. As a contrast, we asked our interviewees which women gave them inspiration as they themselves anticipated getting older. In conclusion, we offer some of their inspirational models.

"My mother is eighty-two and I'd love you to meet her. She's interested in people, aware, fully alive in every way." (*Doreen*)

"A friend who's eighty-six; she's intelligent and great fun. She's always living now, interested in everybody." (*Geraldine*)

"The aunt of a friend; she has immense gaiety and vitality. Very independent—has a lot of courage—she's ninety-two." (*Anne*)

"My mother's a lovely lady; she's eighty-four; she goes to concerts every week. She's always winning prizes for flower arranging." (*Brenda*)

"I hope I will keep an open mind and be as young mentally as my friend is at eighty. She's still whizzing all around visiting everyone. She goes to the theatre, plays tennis, and dresses beautifully." (*Mary*)

"My grandmother was a Cherokee Indian. She got married for the fifth time when she was seventy-nine. She divorced her husband two years later because she refused to get up and milk the cows at five in the morning. She kept the surnames of all her husbands, so at the end of her life, on her gravestone she had this great long list of names." (*Lisa*)

"I listened to a woman in her late seventies lecturing at a conference recently. She was one of the key speakers. Intellectually very sharp, very slim, and kind of tough. I liked that. And my mother, who's in her late seventies now, because she relishes and savors her life. She chooses when she uses her energy; she can be very energetic and then flop out and do nothing when she wants to." (*Bea*)

Afterword

HISTORICALLY, the menopause is a modern phenomenon. Four hundred years ago the average life expectancy for a woman was thirty years. By the beginning of this century it had increased to fifty years. Today a woman in this part of the world has an average life expectancy of seventy-five, so now she faces the prospect of living approximately one third of her life after her reproductive life is over.

This must pose a problem to those who insist that a woman's biology is her sole destiny. If maternity is a woman's sole life purpose, how can one account for her outliving her "usefulness" by twenty-five years? Maybe this paradox underlies the universal and total neglect of menopause as an important rite of passage, since no one can decide what happens after the transition.

There is a cross-cultural belief that a woman loses her womanhood when she stops menstruating. In some societies this means that older women are then able to participate in social and community activities with men, whereas this was denied them when they were menstruating.

But what does it mean for women of the Western world?

It's true that we face change and uncertainty, but also we face an exciting and interesting challenge.

Homeopathic Materia Medica of Menopausal Symptoms

USE the following guidelines:

1. Read through the symptoms listed under each remedy. The ones emphasized in italic type are the clearest guide.

2. In the event that two remedies appear to fit, look closely at *all* the symptoms before making a choice. You can purchase a remedy and try one at a time. Give it a chance to work before abandoning it and trying your second choice. If the remedy doesn't act within 24 hours, it's the wrong remedy, so there's no point in repeating it.

3. Use remedies in potencies of 6x (3c) to 60x (30c) only, starting with 6x (3c) and increasing to 60x (30c). The dose at a potency of 6x (3c) may be repeated four times daily for four days to start with. If after this time no improvement is noticed, the remedy is incorrectly matched. Another remedy may now be selected.

4. If improvement occurs, do not repeat the dose unless there is a relapse.

5. If the low potency works and needs to be repeated, do so at decreasing intervals of time to maintain effectiveness.

6. The 60x (30c) potency is used as a single dose and is repeated on demand.

7. The more severe the symptoms, the more often the medicine should be repeated. As improvement occurs, reduce the frequency. Close observation is the best way to tell when to repeat the medicine.

8. Remedies do not act in the stomach but in the mouth. So don't swallow the tablet or pill; suck it slowly. Do not interfere with the subtlety of the remedy by eating, drinking, or smoking within twenty minutes before or after taking the remedy.

9. It is a good plan to give up coffee (or substitute a decaffeinated or herbal roast drink) while taking homeopathic remedies. If your remedy is nux vomica or ignatia, it is absolutely essential that you give up coffee.

10. Store the remedies away from heat, light, or aromatic substances.

We would again like to emphasize the importance of matching *all* symptoms in *one* category for that remedy to be effective. If you do not find a match, you may prefer to consult a homeopath or herbalist instead of, or as well as, buying a remedy from the store.

The following are fifteen of the more common remedies. All have symptoms of flushing heat (hot flushes).

Lachesis

Flushing, sweating, burning sensation at the top of the head.
Symptoms worse immediately after awakening from sleep (and also just before going to sleep).
External pressure (even of clothing, bed linen) *intolerable*, especially around the neck.
Melancholic mood, gloomy, despairing (intensely religious).
Irritable, ready to jump down people's throats.

Talkative (others cannot get a word in).
May become jealous and suspicious.

Sepia

Flushes with weakness and sweating (but at other times chilly)
Exhaustion: everything is too much effort.
Indifferent to those who were formerly closest and best loved.
Anger, especially when contradicted.
Aversion to sex.
Weeping mood, especially when comparing present state to her
     happier past self. Self-pity and resentment.
Backache and weakness in small of back.
Sensation of *dragging and bearing down* in pelvic area.
Leukorrhea (vaginal discharge), yellow and profuse. Itching
     vagina.
Nausea, especially in the morning; finding the smell of cooking
     particularly unpleasant.

Pulsatilla

Weepy and sad, feels as if she were forsaken, feels alone.
Feeling dependent, craving love and support.
Moods can change in an instant: weepy one moment, happy and gay
     the next.
Irritable and touchy, easily slighted; suspicious.
Flushes (and mood) *better when outdoors*, and benefits from fresh
     air in general.
Feels that she will die if cooped up in a stuffy room.
Cannot tolerate pork or pastry, finds both nauseating.

Nux vomica

Flushes and burning sensation, especially of the face, yet body
     may remain *icy cold*.
Backache, worse in lower back.

Frequent waking from 3 a.m. onward with dreams full of business, bustle, and hurry. Cramps in legs.

Arms, hands, and legs go numb, with sensation of pins and needles.

Nausea, with sensation of weight in stomach. Stomach cramps.

Constipation with ineffectual urging.

Itching of anus. Hemorrhoids.

Intensely irritable, fault-finding. May hold back anger, but the feeling inside is explosive.

Intolerant of noises, strong odors, bright lights.

Ignatia

Nervousness; introspective, *irritable. Hysterical.* Silent brooding. *Sighing.*

Contradictory symptoms. Numbness of various parts.

Sensation of *lump in throat.*

Violent yawning, yet very light sleep. Jerking of limbs before falling asleep.

Constipation with painful *constriction of rectum* after stool.

Sinking sensation in stomach, which is not relieved by eating.

Valeriana

Flushes with heat and sweating, especially on face.

Changeable moods. Hysterical.

Easily irritated by others' comments. Tremulous feelings.

Sleeplessness with itching and muscular spasms.

Sulfur

Violent flushes and sweating, which may smell offensive, like garlic.

Worse at night and for the warmth of bed.

Hot soles of feet and hot hands. Heat or pressure at top of the head.

Redness of mouth, anus, and vagina. *Itching.*

Very thirsty. Sinking feeling at 11 a.m.
Irritable and depressed.
May be egocentric, argumentative.

Ferrum metallicum

Florid and healthy looking, red cheeks, yet exhausted. Red
cheeks, yet mucus membranes are pallid (*anemic*). Sudden
flushes of heat to face and chest. Sweating. Exhausted by any
effort, even speaking and walking.

Helonias

Weakness and dragging weight felt in pelvic area.
Backache and exhaustion.
Womb feels heavy and enlarged.
Itching vagina.

Kali carbonicum

Palpitations (pulse weak and rapid).
Weakness, especially felt in small of back and backs of legs.
Chilly, cannot tolerate drafts.
Sweating easily upon slightest exertion.
Worst time at 2 a.m. "Sour" stomach, regurgitations, bloating.
Indecisive character, easily muddled, yet desires order around
her, committed to a strong sense of right and wrong.

Sulphuricum acidicum

Flushes followed by sweating and trembling, especially in the
evenings and when exercising.
Great weakness.
Very hurried feeling.

Jaborandi

Flushes and sudden profuse *sweating*.
Salivation.

Sanguinaria

Flushes with *redness and burning of cheeks*.
Burning in soles of feel and in palms (symptoms as indicated for
    Sulfur).
Rheumatic complaints in neck, *right shoulder*, and left hip.

Cimicifuga (Actafa racemosa)

Rheumatic and nervous complaints. Flushing and perspiration.
Pains resemble electric shocks. Opening and closing sensation at
    the top of the head.
Stiffness and pain in neck, back, hips, and thighs.
Aching and heaviness in limbs, and in pelvic area.
Depression, as if enveloped in a dark cloud.
Irritable and sighing, petulant and cross.
Talkative and restless.

Aurum metallicum

Palpitations.
Most profound depression with *thoughts of suicide*.
Feeling cut off from love, joy, and light in subjects who have a
    highly evolved conscience; perfectionists.

Further Reading

Boston Women's Health Book Collective. *Our Bodies, Ourselves*, 2nd ed. New York: Simon and Schuster, 1979.

Budoff, Penny Wise, MD. *No More Hot Flashes and Other Good News*. New York: G. P. Putnam's Sons, 1983.

Clay, Vidal S. *Women: Menopause and Middle Age*. Pittsburgh: Know, Inc., 1977.

Greenwood, Sadja, MD. *Menopause, Naturally*. San Francisco: Volcano Press, 1984.

Masters, W., and Johnson, V. "Human Sexual Response: The Aging Female and the Aging Male," in *Middle Age and Aging*. Chicago: University of Chicago Press, 1968.

National Women's Health Network. *Menopause Resource Guide*. Washington, DC: National Women's Health Network.

Reitz, Rosetta. *Menopause: A Positive Approach*. Radnor, PA: Chilton Books, 1977; New York: Penguin, 1979.

Rose, Louise, ed. *The Menopause Book*. New York: Hawthorn Books, 1977.

Seaman, Barbara, and Seaman, Gideon, *Women and the Crisis in Sex Hormones*. New York: Rawson Associates, 1977; New York: Bantam Books, 1978.

Smith, Trevor, MD. *Homeopathic Medicine for Women*. Rochester, VT: Healing Arts Press, 1988.

Treben, Maria. *Health from God's Garden*. Rochester, VT: Healing Arts Press, 1988.

Weideger, Paula. *Menstruation and Menopause: The Physiology and Psychology, the Myth and the Reality*, rev. ed. New York: Dell Publishing, 1977.

Westcott, Patsy and Black, Leyardia, ND. *Alternative Health Care for Women*. Rochester, VT: Healing Arts Press, 1988.

Index

A

abnormal bleeding, 18
aching muscles, 28
adrenal gland, role of, 7, 10
aging, 97–101
alternative treatment for menopause, 69–75
amenorrhea, 40
androgen, 7, 9, 10
androstenedione, 10

B

bladder problems, 26
bleeding, abnormal, 18
bleeding, irregular, 15, 16, 17, 18, 20
bone density, impact of menopause on, 13, 29–30, 64, 65
breasts, impact of menopause on, 8, 13, 17, 20
brittle bone disease, *see* osteoporosis

M

male "menopause" (climacteric), 90–96
men, and the menopause, 90–96
menopausal depression, 31–33, 49
menopause,
    aching muscles and, 28
    aging and, 97–101
    average age at last period, 5, 6
    bladder, impact on, 26
    bone density, impact on, 13, 29–30, 64, 65
    breasts, impact on, 8, 9, 13, 17
    contraception and, 38–41
    definitions of, 5
    depression and, 31–33
    diagnosis of, 15–18, 49, 50
    diet, role of, 77–81
    eczema and, 27, 28
    exercise and, 81–83
    headaches and, 25
    hot flushes and night sweats and, 21–24, 40, 49, 61, 62
    indications of, 15–18
    insomnia and, 27
    male "menopause" (climacteric), comparison with, 90–96
    menstrual irregularity and, 15–18
    men's reactions to, 90–96
    osteoporosis and, 29, 30, 64, 65
    palpitations and, 25
    premature, 18, 19
    sexuality and, 36–46
    skin changes and, 27, 28
    smoking and, 6, 76
    stress and, 34–35
    treatment with herbal medicine, 73–75
    treatment with homeopathy, 69–75, 103–108
    treatment with hormone replacement therapy (HRT), 50, 54–68
menstrual cycle, 6, 7, 10–12
menstrual irregularity, 15–18
mineral supplements in diet, 80–81

N

night sweats, 21–24. *See also* hot flushes